Integrated Ongoing Neurological Support in the Community

MAKING A DIFFERENCE

Edited by
Eleanor Kinnear
David Beales
Alan Paton

Independently Published

First Published 2023

The Editors: makingadifference4neuro@gmail.com

Contents

Foreword

The National Health Service (NHS) provides time-limited periods of outpatient therapy to neurological patients after which the patient is usually discharged, even whilst having persisting or deteriorating disabilities. There is often a delay of several weeks or even months from referral to the patient receiving an assessment by the NHS neurologist or movement disorder specialist, speech and language therapy, physiotherapist, or occupational therapist.

Presently neurological services in the United Kingdom are not integrated and there is little interaction between patients' hospital-based clinicians, their general practitioner and community-based therapy services. This situation is compounded by the shortage of neurologists in the UK and the very brief period of training in neurology that medical students receive in their clinical years at medical school, which currently averages just over two weeks. The needs of the patient's carer are rarely considered, and the patient and their family have to negotiate the complex world of social support, both financial and emotional.

This book shows what might be a difficult and deteriorating life for those with long-standing neurological conditions and their carers, can be avoided. There is great scope to improve the quality of life through patient centred integrated neurological rehabilitation and support in the community. A prime objective is to prevent crises, rather than just responding to them, by minimising a patient's disability and social handicap, even when they are progressive, and optimising their function.

Key elements in achieving this are a multi-disciplinary team, with different skills, working with a patient to create a personalised program, an ongoing health record, and greater knowledge for the patient of their condition enabling self-help side by side with hospital provision. The book provides a better understanding of neurological conditions and how best to plan, act, and reach optimal function.

This not only improves the lives of individuals but significantly diminishes unnecessary hospital re-admissions from preventable crises and saves the NHS significant sums of money.

An excellent example of what can be achieved is given by Integrated Neurological Services (INS), a medical charity operating in the London boroughs of Hounslow and Richmond upon Thames, mentioned in this book, and to which I have referred many patients

Dr Peter Bain MBBS MA (Oxon) MD FRCP.

Reader in the Department of Brain Sciences at Imperial College London, and Honorary Consultant in Clinical Neurology, Charing Cross Hospital, Imperial College Healthcare NHS Trust

Introduction

Most of us will know a friend or relative with a neurological condition or may want to look at ways to prevent or manage such an occurrence. Over 5% of UK adults – nearly three million people – have a neurological condition; Stroke, Traumatic Brain Injury, Parkinson's disease, Multiple Sclerosis (MS), Brain Tumour, Motor Neurone disease, and many others.

There is huge scope and need to complement the NHS. Following the initial diagnosis and treatment of a condition people return home with most support being provided by a family member. They have to make the best of it for the rest of their life and this is a huge challenge. Without the right expertise to hand or understanding of their condition it is the case that they will often have to call again on hospital or GP help and their quality of life is poor.

The right support, therapeutic and social, can make all the difference. Prime objectives of this book are to show people with neurological conditions that their quality of life can be improved and to show how the right support might be most effectively organised and delivered.

There is a great amount of information which is often complex and detailed so great care has been taken to help the reader. The book is divided into four parts.

PART 1 summarises the national situation and highlights the findings and recommendations of the Health Foundation and the MS Society concerning ongoing support, self-help, and continued multi-disciplinary rehabilitation in the community.

PART 2 gives the personal accounts of people with neurological conditions, their carers, and supporting volunteers, covering time of diagnosis, how matters developed, and the situation today. It shows how people benefit from a greater knowledge of their condition, self-help, and integrated, ongoing, local support.

PART 3 covers advances in rehabilitation, how issues can be addressed and summarises best practice based on the lessons of experience .

PART 4 describes the "why" and "how" of the creation of a charity providing integrated and ongoing neurological support in the community.

The book is a "short read". It is divided into numerous but brief chapters and sections, clearly named in an explanatory style, making it easy to follow and absorb.

~~~~~

All the proceeds from the sales of this book are donated to the medical charity Integrated Neurological Services (INS). https://www.ins.org.uk/

Acknowledgements

A special thank you to all those with neurological conditions, their carers, and supporting volunteers, who have made an enormous contribution to this book. What they have to say is the heart of it.

Thank you: Jackie Dee, Anne, Imelda O'Shaughnessy, Anne Thomsett, Hugh Fells, Maggie Hughes, Julie Burgess, Cia Van der Sluis, Sara Challice, Bindu Thakrar, Bharti Patel, Jon McPherson, Nick Berners-Price, Stuart Banks, Keith Severs, Pritam Brar, Anne Foulds, Alexander Reed, Kate Hodgkinson, Janet Holmes, Daphne Jowit, Caroline Hill, Carol Williams.

Thanks also for help on the photographic side to Sally Faulkner, Mark Doust, and Caroline Walker.
~~~~~

Chapter Authors & Book Editors

Eleanor (Ellie) Kinnear is a physiotherapist whose journey into neurology has been inspired by her experience of meeting young people with a stroke in their early 20s. She has been involved in research into people with Parkinson's, Stroke and learning difficulty. Through attending a lecture she was introduced to the Conductive Education approach for rehabilitation of neurological conditions. This influenced how the integrated neurological charity she founded evolved; truly holistic, involving home visits, group work, activities and outings with support for the family carers.

David Beales became a general practitioner after training in rheumatology and rehabilitation at Guys and Kings College Hospitals. David combined general practice with five hospital sessions in acute care and rehabilitation as hospital practitioner and acting consultant in elderly care. In 1991 he founded The Cirencester and District Charitable Trust to finance anticipatory health care for older people called Stay Well 75+ In 2000 he was invited to become Chief Medical Officer at The Bristol Cancer Help Centre and trained in Mind-Body medicine. He has contributed to five books and given numerous workshops and presentations. He developed Parkinson's disease, with Consultant Neurologist confirmation, in August 2017. He is learning to self-care and remains well.

Sara Challice gave up her career as a graphic designer with a large London investment company to care for her husband for 13 years after he was diagnosed with a brain tumour. Following a stroke, he became bedbound and needed full-time nursing care; due to the pressure, Sara became both mentally and physically unwell. She then found new strategies to regain her health and enjoy life again, even whilst caring for a terminally ill husband. Sara also got involved with local and national charities and became a trustee for INS (Integrated Neurological Services).

Alan Paton is a Friend of INS. He is retired and was the founder of a publishing and seminars company mainly concerned with Internet technology and electronic publishing. He has written and published several books on historical subjects.

PART 1

MEETING THE CHALLENGES

Chapter 1
The Nature & Challenges of Neurological Conditions

Neurological Conditions

A neurological condition is a disease, illness or trauma that affects the central or peripheral nervous system. Examples of symptoms include paralysis, tremor, cognitive difficulties, muscle weakness, poor coordination, loss of sensation, seizures, confusion, pain and altered levels of consciousness.

There are more than 600 recognised conditions. The table below shows some of the most well-known and their prevalence in the UK.

Neurological Condition	**UK Prevalence 2022**
Traumatic Brain Injury	1,300,000
Stroke	1,290,000
Parkinson's disease	145,000
Multiple Sclerosis (MS)	130,000
Post-Polio syndrome	120,000
Brain Tumours	102,000
Cerebral Palsy	30,000
Huntington's disease	8,000
Motor neurone disease	5,000

Source: Editor's estimates based on statistics published by the Neurological Alliance, [1] the Stroke Association, Parkinson's UK, and the MS Society.

Long-term neurological conditions can be broadly categorised as follows:

Sudden onset conditions, for example acquired brain injury, stroke, or spinal cord injury, followed by a partial recovery.

Intermittent and unpredictable conditions, for example epilepsy, certain types of headaches or early multiple sclerosis, where relapses and remissions lead to marked variation in the care needed.

Progressive conditions, for example motor neurone disease, Parkinson's disease or later stages of multiple sclerosis, where progressive deterioration in neurological function leads to increasing dependence on help and care from others. For some conditions (e.g. motor neurone disease) deterioration can be rapid.

Stable neurological conditions, but with changing needs due to development or ageing, for example post-polio syndrome or cerebral palsy in adults.

Consequences for People

Neurological conditions affect people of all ages, ethnicity groups, and social and economic backgrounds. Sadly, neurological conditions have not gained the high profile of other diseases, for instance, more women die of neurological conditions than breast cancer.

- Patients with neurological conditions have the lowest health related quality of life of any long-term condition.

- A huge amount of pressure is placed on the carer where often they may be elderly and infirm themselves and have no awareness of the condition or its implications.

- The isolation and loneliness they suffer is further exacerbated when speech is badly affected and their difficulties with mobility lead to decline longer term.

- The likelihood of having a mental health condition alongside their neurological one is higher for neurology patients than for other long-term conditions.

- Aside from their debilitating health, they are left to navigate the complexities of benefits and social services alone. There is no ongoing support. This can cause endless frustration, worry and despair.

Many people with neurological conditions have worsening symptoms which lead to increasing difficulties with simple everyday activities – dressing, walking, talking, eating, socialising with family and friends and engaging in the world outside the home. In addition, there can be side effects from medication and the presence of continuous pain. Their world becomes smaller as their physical independence reduces, alongside cognitive and sensory decline in many cases. Cultural, language and educational barriers can exacerbate these challenges and increase isolation and depression.

> *"For me the disease is totally unpredictable, meaning I suddenly freeze, movements are slow, horrendous back pain, tremor, I basically have no control and at times through the day, I cannot stand, walk or even keep my balance."*
> Jon on Parkinson's disease, 49 years old

Some will have to face the inevitable loss of financial independence. They are left with no option but the reality of accepting social benefits, and many may struggle to navigate the practicalities of accessing benefits, made even more difficult if their communication is impaired too; often a loved one will have to give up their job or independence to become a carer, so two lives are negatively impacted.

The physical impact of long-term neurological conditions affects each individual differently. Many conditions cause degeneration over many years and can cause problems with coordination, vision, weakness, fatigue, sexual function, bladder and bowel issues and cognitive problems to name a few.

Life will change drastically and will present the newly diagnosed individual with an array of issues that need to be addressed immediately, and some issues that will need to be addressed in the medium and long-term.

Questions they need to face are how will they be able to support themselves physically and financially? Many will lose their driving licence and will be faced with transport challenges. Many will face an array of restrictions which mean they will become socially isolated. Some will experience language impairment, so will face difficulties with telephone banking or being able to ask simple questions and understand simple answers or directions. Their lives will often be transformed from being independent to being heavily reliant on others and this can be extremely frustrating for them. Not everyone will have the benefit of someone to care for them or have family nearby or living with them.

Their partners/carers also face life-changing situations in their unexpected role as a carer for which they are unprepared and to which they need time to adjust. Carers will have little background knowledge of neurological conditions, how to support the individual or even what degeneration can be expected. Physically they may develop injuries such as bad backs and psychological stress and depression are common.

Acute Treatment and What Follows

• After providing acute hospital care, the NHS can only fund short-term limited support. It neither helps people to reach and maintain their potential for as long as possible assisting them to remain in their occupations or assist them to find an alternative one, nor does it assist when there is a deterioration with very complicated cases especially when the family care giver can no longer cope, thus avoiding a crisis intervention.

• A life devastated upon diagnosis, only to be discharged from the healthcare system after just six weeks rehabilitation.

• Individuals are left to cope on their own, often to stagnate until they decline, just waiting for the next medical episode to occur, which will often debilitate them further.

Patients with neurological conditions are not being supported on a long-term basis by the NHS. The same is true of council social care except for the few councils that fund voluntary organisations such as INS [See below] and the Stroke Association.

Andrew Marr, the well-known TV presenter, had a stroke. He found that after being given therapy twice a day as an in-patient in hospital, he was provided with therapy once a week when he was discharged home. Typically, the NHS only funds a few sessions when people return home and patients are discharged from the healthcare system after just six weeks rehabilitation. He was lucky, he could afford private therapy to help his ongoing improvement for increasing independence. This demonstrates a lack in helping people reach and maintain their potential and be as independent for as long as possible.

People with a neurological condition often enter a loop of diagnosis, care in hospital, discharge into community service, discharge home, crisis or an event leading to readmission to acute services.

> *"After hospital Parminder was given physio for about four or five weeks. Then that was it. You are left to your own devices. They said to us, 'You don't understand you have to live with this now'. I felt very frustrated, and it broke my heart. INS helped a lot. They helped her use her right hand again and start writing. We can call any time if we need more help. INS are so helpful."*
> Mr H and his Wife, Stroke Client

This leads to an ever-increasing burden on:

- Social services
- GP services
- and bed blocking in hospital.

NHS data shows that neurological conditions are involved in the majority of bed blocking patients - either as a primary or co-condition. Yet only one in five Clinical Commissioning Groups (CCGs) have assessed prevalence and costs locally and little data is routinely collected nationally.

> *"Rehabilitation in the UK is a Cinderella service and the cost in human and money terms is enormous."*
> Nicholas Boyle, Consultant Surgeon, Times letters 08/08/2018
>
> *"Clear local care pathways for patients with common neurology conditions have often been neglected, resulting in fragmented, inefficient and ineffective care. Data on CCG spending for emergency care for these common conditions shows considerable opportunities to improve care at lower cost."*
> David Bateman MD FRCP, Consultant Neurologist

A Major Problem – Vital Facts and Figures

According to the 2020 GP Patient survey, 18% of patients with a neurological condition had an unplanned stay in hospital over the past year – this is nearly twice the rate for all people with a long-term condition (10%). [2] [3]

It is well documented that for people with ambulatory care sensitive conditions – such as epilepsy or ataxia or other long-term neurological conditions – an A&E attendance or emergency hospital admission represents a gap elsewhere in the health system. These attendances and emergency admissions are an avoidable expense and place individuals where they least want to be.

Something Can be Done

Confidence and Self-Management

Recent research by the Health Foundation revealed that 690,000 A&E attendances could be avoided if people were supported to better manage their long-term conditions. (This covers all long-term conditions, not just neurological conditions.)

> The research looks at how well patients feel able to manage their long-term conditions. **It finds that those who felt most confident and able to manage their condition and keep themselves well had 38% fewer emergency admissions and 32% fewer A&E attendances than those who felt least able.** They also had 18% fewer general practice appointments. [4]
>
> **If patients were better supported to manage their long-term conditions – for example, through health coaching, peer support or greater access to apps that help people to manage symptoms and avoid deteriorations – this could lead to a reduction in emergency admissions to hospital, A&E attendances and GP appointments.**
>
> In the best-case scenario, if the patients who currently feel least able to manage their conditions were supported to manage their conditions as well as those who feel most able, this could prevent 436,000 emergency admissions to hospital and 690,000 attendances at A&E each year. **This equates to 7% of the total number of emergency admissions and 6% of A&E attendances in England each year.**
>
> The research, which looked at levels of knowledge, skill and confidence in self-management for over 9,000 adults with long-term conditions, is the first NHS study to demonstrate a link between self-management and patients' use of health services across both primary and secondary care. As well as having fewer emergency admissions and A&E attendances, the patients who felt most able to manage their health had 18% fewer general practice appointments.
>
> In the study, just 13% of patients felt knowledgeable about their health condition and confident to plan and manage their care. While almost a quarter (22%) were likely to feel overwhelmed by the

demands of their long-term condition and not take an active role in their own care.

Over the last 12 years, the number of emergency hospital admissions in England has increased by 42% from 4.25 million in 2006/07 to 6.02 million in 2017/18. Over 60% of patients admitted to hospital as an emergency have one or more long-term health conditions such as asthma, diabetes or a mental illness.

Sarah Deeny, Assistant Director of Data Analytics at the Health Foundation, said: *Patients with long-term conditions manage the majority of their care, spending less than 1% of their time in contact with a health professional.* ***Supporting these patients to develop the necessary skills, knowledge and confidence to manage their health as effectively as possible is critical to helping them stay well and could help reduce the need for a vast number of emergency admissions, A&E attendances and GP appointments.***

To ease pressure on services and improve patients' quality of life, national policy makers and the local NHS must take action now to support people to better manage their long-term conditions. This should include NHS England prioritising support for self-management in the long-term plan for the NHS.

Health Foundation, August 2018

Integration and Support in the Community

In October 2021, the MS Society published the report *Neurology now - The case for a new approach to neurology services,* summarising its recent studies and latest research. [5]

With MS for example, people live with the condition for many years and good care can require up to a dozen services working together. It's the kind of condition that requires long-term, joined-up thinking across the NHS and other systems, offering a template for more integrated care across the whole population.

.... There's strong evidence showing continued, coordinated multi-disciplinary rehabilitation in the community improves long-term outcomes and can help to reduce hospital re-admissions. Self-management and preventative measures supported by trained healthcare professionals are invaluable to people with neurological conditions to prevent decline and ill-health.

.... Our overarching recommendation is for all Governments of the four nations to develop and resource national plans to restore and improve neurology services by working with neurological charities and patients.

.... NHS bodies should explore opportunities to partner with charity and third sector organisations locally to offer truly joined-up care for people with neurological conditions.

MS Society, October 2021

To Sum Up!

- The NHS doesn't provide long-term support to people with neurological conditions!

- Consequently, after initial treatment people with neurological conditions often require unplanned or emergency hospital treatment; twice as much as those with other long-term conditions. There are similar unplanned demands on GP services.

- Those with long-term conditions who are more confident about managing their condition themselves, require far less emergency treatment and are far happier, which is also important for the well-being of their family.

- Integrated support and self-management are vital.

- Great benefits can be achieved by services that complement the NHS

Making a Difference – Complementing the NHS

The next PART of the book contains 23 personal accounts of people with neurological conditions, those who care for them, and volunteers who help support them, describing how their life has been affected, the problems they have encountered, and how they have been involved in and benefited from integrated and ongoing local support.

Most accounts involve Integrated Neurological Services (INS), a medical charity based in the London boroughs of Richmond and Hounslow. [https://www.ins.org.uk/] INS refers to those it supports as its "Clients". It employs a multi-disciplinary team providing physiotherapy, occupational therapy, speech and language therapy, social work support, and classes such as creative writing, and a Mind, Body, and Spirit group.

First, some very brief extracts of what Clients and Carers have to say about some of the benefits

Jackie Dee – Stroke Client

... an occupational therapist took me out to teach me how to use an escalator in Dickens & Jones. We went up and down, again and again on the escalators, which made such a difference to me as I had been so scared. Now I could go independently to see my daughter by the Underground – this was some five years after I had had my stroke.

Anne – Stroke Client

At first, I attended the exercise class which helped physically and later joined other classes. All this helped both mentally and physically and I made new friends. Very reassuring knowing where to find information and have someone to talk to where they had time to answer any questions and check progress.

.... Using the treadmill was brilliant. It meant I could walk faster than outdoors, total support from the handrails, less risk of tripping and help on hand should it be needed. It meant I could concentrate on the way I walked, more upright and looking ahead instead of looking where to place my feet.

Bindu Thakrar – PD Client

.... just what I needed as we were a group of clients in the same boat although at different stages, different symptoms and different medications. The group forum allowed for all of us to share experiences which gave me a lot of information and insight of what was to come and how I may be affected by Parkinson's going forward.

.... The groups which have especially helped me are sleep management, speech and language therapy, mind, body, and spirit, and the exercise session, which all include time to discuss problems with an opportunity to share information and advice.

.... I have gained a lot of knowledge about my condition and been supported by professional qualified people in a friendly and caring way. Also very helpful is sharing experiences with others in the same boat and making friends that can relate to my issues and my feelings and be very supportive in ways that family and friends aren't always able to.

Bharti Patel – PD Client
.... If I get emotional then my tremor increases, but when I took the Mindfulness Meditation group I felt much calmer. I now practise this on my own. I find the staff friendly and I feel safe.

Stuart Banks – Carer for Gail Banks – MS Client
.... As well as regularly assessing Gail at home, they looked closely at what my needs were. They taught me how I could cope better, explained the nature of the condition that Gail had. Everything from physio techniques, speech and language therapy; a journey that helped me to help Gail and helped me to realise that I have a life.

Keith Severs – Carer for Pat Severs – PD Client
I feel very strongly that Pat, without INS's help and support, would not have coped with PD as well as she actually managed. This is underlined by the contrast between her progress and that of her sister Joyce, who also had PD. Joyce did not have the good fortune to live in the INS catchment area, so had no therapy and only minimal support; her decline was very much faster than Pat's.

Pritam Brar – Carer for Gurdev Brar – PD Client
1 Exercise for my husband to control his Parkinson's deterioration by trained therapists and staff who are so helpful and caring.

He was able to communicate with people in a similar condition. He looked forward to meeting his Exercise group every week. This enabled him to get ready in the morning, travelling by car, the whole day became exciting, and gaining valuable experience.

2 Support for me as a carer.

I was listened to with empathy and an understanding of how difficult it was for me to cope with my husband's behaviour under the side effects of the drug agonists. I was offered a 12-week counselling with fully experienced therapist. Counselling healed me and got me out of the dark hole I was stuck in for so long that I even forgot how to smile.

Maggie Hughes – Carer for Trevor Hughes – Stroke Client
Having been told that he would never be able to walk after leaving hospital Ellie and Judit set about changing that way of thinking. Through Judit's programme she encouraged him to use his paralysed side, to stand

and walk using a ladder chair, eventually leading him to walking with a narrow-based quad stick and close supervision.

REFERENCES

[1] *Neuro Numbers 2019*, Neurological Alliance https://www.neural.org.uk/wp-content/uploads/2021/04/neuro-numbers-2019-1.pdf

[2] *The long-term plan for the NHS: Getting it right for neurology patients*, Neurological Alliance, 2018 https://www.neural.org.uk/assets/pdfs/2018-08-long-term-plan-for-nhs.pdf

[3] *GP Patient Survey*, Ipsos MORI https://gp-patient.co.uk/

[4] Sarah Deeny, Ruth Thorlby, Adam Steventon, *Briefing: Reducing emergency admissions: Unlocking the potential of people to better manage their long-term conditions*, The Health Foundation, August 2018 https://www.health.org.uk/publications/reducing-emergency-admissions-unlocking-the-potential-of-people-to-better-manage-their-long-term-conditions

690,000 A&E attendances could be avoided, The Health Foundation, August 2018 https://www.health.org.uk/news-and-comment/news/690000-ae-attendances-could-be-avoided-if-people

[5] *Neurology now - The case for a new approach to neurology services*, MS Society, October 2021, https://www.mssociety.org.uk/what-we-do/news/neurology-report

~~~~~
~~~~~

PART 2

REAL-LIFE EXPERIENCE

Chapter 2
Real-Life Experience – Stroke, Brain Injury, & Tumours

CLIENTS

Jackie Dee – Stroke Client – My Stroke Victory

I was cleaning and went into the kitchen - and I remember nothing more! I half-heard my mobile ring but I couldn't get to it. The thing I heard next was Georgina, my daughter. Oh, what a mess she must have found! I had been sick three times, so I learnt some time later. And I had been lying there for 28 hours!

I went in an ambulance to Kingston hospital, went through A&E but didn't wake up. Then I awoke in bed, I don't know when, and Georgina asked me something, and I answered her. She didn't understand a word I said, which she told me a couple of months later.

My other daughter, Christina, was riding a bicycle for charity in Borneo, and my brother and sister-in-law were on holiday on a cruise. But when they got back they rushed to my side, with my sister-in-law (a nurse) taking control.

The Start of My Journey

I spent three weeks in hospital, during which time I had a couple of pulmonary embolisms (a blocked blood vessel in the lungs which can be life-threatening if not treated quickly), and some help from the physiotherapists and speech therapists. Then I went in an ambulance to my sister-in-law's home.

I paid for two physiotherapists, an occupational therapist, a speech therapist, and some others, and five weeks later I was just about able to walk for about five feet before collapsing! My speech was much improved, going up from about 40% to about 75%, and I was shown how to try to walk up-stairs, and I thought I would never do it! But I did!

I went home for Christmas, then went to the Wolfson Neurorehabilitation Centre in Wimbledon at the beginning of the year. I was in there for three months, doing so very much, I don't know how I did it! There were physiotherapist doing brilliantly, occupational therapists showing ironing, kitchen things, and art, which was fabulous, and I drew with my left hand a couple in "brass". Brilliant!

The head physiotherapist was taking me back to my room, and she said that she wished she could help with my right arm but couldn't - that was the first time I believed my right arm was too bad to be of any use!

Back Home

At home I had a physiotherapist and occupational therapist for nine weeks and then she told me I was on my own. She asked me what I'd like to do, and I said art, to which she said "lovely", and then I asked "could I do Pilates?", and she quietly said "Oh, I don't think so, dear".

I thought to myself, "just you wait and see"! I went to Richmond College, signed in for art and Pilates, and I'm still doing art and Pilates! This was just a year after my stroke!

I was told to have some driving lessons and then I would have my driving licence again, and then I got a car with facilities. I took trips to the gym, Pilates, art, and the theatre and cinema, not to mention my family and friends. Sometime in 2005 I was referred to INS.

Involvement with INS

I found the people at INS amazing! They did some movements, talk and tea with a man doing our exercises each week! Also, an INS occupational therapist, Kara Dunn, took me out to teach me how to use an escalator in Dickens & Jones. We went up and down, again and again on the escalators, which made such a difference to me as I had been so scared. Now I could go independently to see my daughter by the Underground – this was some five years after I had had my stroke.

We have St George's medical students come to INS and I often took part in telling them the story of my stroke when I also told them of my twice broken arm! I was seeing Georgina, my daughter, on the second Mother's Day after my stroke, and fell over and broke my arm; the ambulance took me to Kingston Hospital, when I was with the radiologist, she said as she looked at the X-ray that I had broken my arm before. To which I replied that "I hadn't" and she said "Yes, you have because I can see it". Then I realised that that was the reason my arm had hurt so much when I was first in hospital with my stroke. Nobody had checked it! Well, I guess I was rather ill! The students now know such things happen and can use that knowledge in their careers.

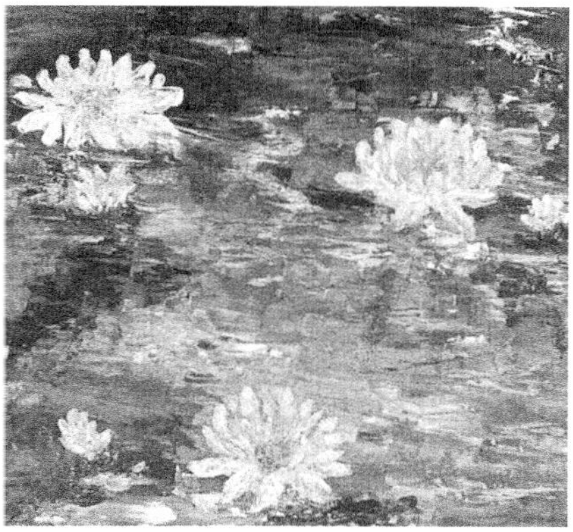

Painting by Jackie

I took part in the Art group in the INS Expanding Horizons Programme when I and others learnt to paint on glass. A selection of glass I painted was exhibited in a church in Barnes and sold for £200. I was delighted to give the money to INS.

12 years after my stroke I have been living on my own, buying all my food, doing my cooking, washing and ironing, a real victory over my stroke. I was still involved with INS and also taking part in collecting money outside Dicken & Jones in Richmond quite a few times over the years and in other fundraising events.

Four years ago, I moved to Lynwood Village for the over 65+, with a swimming pool. There the swimming pool instructor, Lee, taught me how to swim on my back with one arm, which I now do very happily on my own. I have joined an Art group there. We are doing astonishingly well!

So that's my story for the past 18 years, in 2021.

~~~~~

Anne – Stroke Client

It was not obvious that I had stroke, both legs not working properly. My daughter took me to Ashford walk-in. Not sure what it was, they asked my daughter to take me to St Peter's for a CT scan. Their scanner not working so sent back to Ashford by ambulance and back to St Peter's afterwards (no need for blue light they were told). Stroke confirmed and treatment started. Took me to a ward. By this time, I had lost some feeling and movement on left side.

My stay there was fine and eventually they sent me to rehab at Ashford. Very well looked after and helped there.

On discharge went to live with my family in Sunbury until stronger and more able to manage stairs. Someone always on call there, family or retired neighbours. Physio not possible as I live in Hounslow and son in Spelthorne. Physio not able to cross border. When returning home had a few short visits. A few leaflets and checked how I was doing with some new exercises. Felt I was being rushed and questions not answered.
~~~~~

INS Makes a Difference

When I could get into a car one of my best friends picked me up and took me to classes I enjoyed. Whilst attending Tai Chi, I saw an INS occupational therapist (I knew her from Age UK) escorting a gentleman, and she gave me details of INS. It took a while to get the courage to phone and meet new people but I'm so glad I did. Everyone really welcoming with lovely smiles. Not looked back.

At first, I attended the exercise class which helped physically and later joined other classes. All this helped both mentally and physically and I made new friends. Very reassuring knowing where to find information and have someone to talk to where they had time to answer any questions and check progress.

The classes at INS and also for 60+ Hounslow residents, and friends and family, all helped. Hounslow classes were nearer and more accessible. I attended the INS Mind, Body, and Spirit group which I found very relaxing especially the meditation, and I found hearing and discussing various subjects stimulating and uplifting. I also attended the Music group and, until the day changed, gym sessions. Using the treadmill was brilliant. It meant I could walk faster than outdoors, total support from the handrails, less risk of tripping and help on hand should it be needed. It meant I could concentrate on the way I walked, more upright and looking ahead instead of looking where to place my feet.

Loved these sessions but a day change meant clashing with two other activities I regularly attended; both nearer with a small charge or free. It was a very difficult decision. Using the treadmill was brilliant but meant giving up two other activities. Also loved extra activities INS arranged both at INS and other locations, especially a trip to bowling club.

As someone always on the go before the stroke (Tai Chi, yoga, line dance five times a week and exercise classes), INS classes helped me find different interests. Have attended different classes; mindfulness, gardening, creative writing, art, music to name a few and many one offs. Love to try something new. I can't praise INS enough. It really helped.

Had my stroke in 2014 and joined INS sometime in 2015 and am still involved.

~~~~~
~~~~~

Imelda O'Shaughnessy – Stroke Client

Time of Diagnosis

I didn't believe the diagnosis, I wasn't aware of my physical condition, I thought nothing had changed in my life until I couldn't carry out the usual, normal daily tasks. I was angry and frustrated that people were talking at me like a child and talking about me, I kept feeling overwhelmed, crying, unable and wanted to get out/die. It was the first anniversary of my husband's death. My four adult children were devastated.

A Difficult Journey

I had painful gynaecological conditions in addition to stroke conditions that I was slowly becoming more aware of. There were new challenges daily. From being unable to dress myself properly; make the bed; put away the washing; read the calendar or indeed read and write coherently, particularly anything boxed or in a grid. All of the simplest processing and organisational skills were disappearing from my life.

Family and friends were not communicating in a way that I could understand. Most often they misunderstood what I was saying. They were intent on making me listen but I was unable to process the information. They became totally frustrated trying to get me to understand. It made me feel helpless and want to give up. My children were between very frustrated and very frightened for me.

With community support from an occupational therapist, grief counselling, and the Red Cross, I somehow became intent on some sort of recovery. Unfortunately, the time allocated for occupational therapists was running out. The second occupational therapist was about to finish up. My other last and valued support was from the Red Cross.

Then I managed to contact the local Stroke group and was told to come along after Christmas (Dec 2019). I attended the group twice but a few days before the third meeting I was informed there wasn't a place for me after all and I would have to be put on a waiting list. I experienced a depressing sense of rejection because at this time the Stroke group appeared to be the only physical and mental support I could possibly expect.

I was in despair of getting any further help. Although I knew the occupational therapists had signed me up for a couple of things (INS and a return-to-work project). At the time I didn't remember. I didn't know what they were or what they meant. I was confused, unable to process and recall any new information.

My only hope was a vague belief that I might be able to affect a return to work and to driving again. To try and recover some sort of normality.

I felt people were obstructing or preventing me from doing so I hadn't fully accepted my disability (this is the first time I have owned "my disability", admitted it). Mostly I am verbally and physically capable which tends to disguise any disability.

I didn't understand the procedures of sickness and absence from work. I went along with whatever the professionals advised/directed; doctor; consultant; occupational therapist; union; therapist and family. It was an anxious and bewildering time.

INS Gets Things Moving in the Right Direction

Next, a contact from social worker Carol, from INS, brought me great hope. It was a blessing. I was offered a variety of familiar activities I could get involved with, things I related to; arts and craft, music, meeting people, things I could do and be a part of. There were a number of other things also if I needed them.

Then came the lock down. Initially, I had difficulty using my phone and accessing my computer so the likelihood of attending a Zoom meeting was most unlikely. Against hope, I decided to try the Zoom and attend a music meeting. I was very surprised and very pleased with my Zoom success when I was quite low. I had lots of support from Sophie and members of the Music group. A friendship and trust followed almost immediately.

It had been difficult to recover some voice, but I was encouraged by the care and understanding of the group. I was introduced to other groups in INS including the Mind, Body, and Spirit group. This was a huge breakthrough.

INS has saved me from impending clinical depression and probably worse. This with the support of family and good friends has given me hope of a productive future.

~~~~~
~~~~~

CARERS

Anne Thomsett – Carer for Murray Thomsett – Stroke Client

He was taken ill in the evening. I suspected he was having a stroke. Speech slurred. Couldn't move himself. I rang 999 at 8.10pm. Again at 8.25pm when I saw he couldn't move his left side. Again at 8.50pm when still no sign of an ambulance because he was becoming unconscious. An ambulance arrived at 9pm. He was blue lighted to St George's Hospital. It was the longest hours of my life. He remained in ITU there for four weeks. I was told he would never walk again. All staff were very kind and worked hard on him, but I was very bewildered. Most of that time he wasn't aware of anything.

Initial Treatment and Rehabilitation

Eventually he was moved to Kingston Hospital for several weeks before being taken to Queen Mary's for rehab. By then he was able to take notice, but I don't think he really realised how bad he was. Frustrated that he couldn't move himself. Got cross when people didn't let him do as he wanted. They continued to sort out his ability to swallow safely. Gradually he could speak again..... and how! With daily physio they enabled him to sit unsupported for a short period of time and to partially wash and dress himself. He had enough core strength to be able to use a patient turner (rota stand) which made transfers much easier.

However, he had lost the ability to understand cause and effect. He got annoyed that he wasn't allowed to get up out of bed when he chose. Couldn't comprehend he could get hurt. He often got cross with me for not helping him to move about or do things. If I said 'No' he would point out that I had no medical qualifications so what did I know?!

Abrupt Termination of Treatment

Suddenly after about five months in Queen Mary's the social worker (whom I had never met) rang to say that he should leave the hospital ASAP. They had reached the end of the treatment they could give him. I was to find a place in a care home pronto.

I had already started looking for suitable care homes but had not realised there was such urgency. The social worker never made me feel that she was there to help and guide me through the process. She was there to make sure I followed the rules regardless of my situation.

Thankfully, a friend was with me when the call came through. He promptly offered his help. He has a daughter who was a care home manager and another who was a social worker. He himself has a good understanding of finance. What a Godsend! He came with me to meet Murray's allocated social worker and the council finance people. I was very anxious about affording everything and finding out about our entitlements. All I remember the hospital suggesting was that I should contact The Stroke Association. They were only able to offer activities we could join in. Not appropriate at that stage. Anyway, Murray wasn't a 'joiner-in'.

Very Limited Post-Discharge Support

Murray was discharged from hospital to go into a care home, with a package of exercises he should be helped to do, with a promise that he would hear from the community physios and OTs in due course. It was several months before anyone contacted us. Six physio sessions were given. The physio wasn't interested in looking at the carefully prepared package from the hospital. As it had been so long since he had been receiving daily physio they had to start from scratch.

All that had been achieved in hospital had been totally wasted. I was unable to persuade him to do the exercises with me. The care home staff had neither the time nor inclination to do them with him either. He couldn't understand that the exercises would be any help in getting him moving again.

INS Become Involved

After he had been in the care home for about six months (over a year after his stroke) I heard about INS from the relative of one of the residents. At last, here were some people who could help without setting a time limit of six sessions. A physiotherapist from INS took Murray on and gradually got him to sit and even stand and walk a few steps with assistance. He also arranged for the delivery of a patient turner which he taught Murray and the care home staff to use. It made life so much easier for all. Sadly, a year or so later one of the care home staff pushed Murray rather than the turner when moving him. The result was that Murray fell.

The care home then deemed it to be a health and safety issue and refused to let him use it again. After that he was always hoisted and lost his core muscle strength. INS sent a letter to our GP telling them about the incident. INS continued physio for a couple of years but had to stop because Murray stopped cooperating. Murray would never do any exercises between sessions. He really enjoyed his sessions with the INS physiotherapist so it was sad they had to stop. He had progressed so much in the time given to him by INS.

When he left Queen Mary's he had been given a motorised wheelchair as well as a manual one. This gave him a little more independence which he loved. However, he could only use it within the building as his ability to judge distances, especially his left side awareness, had been damaged by the stroke.

Move to Another Care Home and INS Help with Wheelchair

He had to be moved to another care home as the first one could no longer meet his needs (some dementia had set in making him violent occasionally).

The new care home wouldn't allow the motorised wheelchair due to the number of wandering residents in their dementia unit. It became obvious that the manual wheelchair that Murray now had wasn't suitable for him to sit in all day. I was having problems with the Wheelchair department at Queen Mary's in getting a properly supportive manual wheelchair supplied in place of the original. I discussed this with INS. Carol Hopkins kindly sent a letter in support of my request. Finally, they agreed. Thank you Carol and INS!

Problems Caused by Wrong Medication

I suspect that much of Murray's anger and frustration stemmed from the fact that he was never out of pain. Due to muscle wastage he lived with a left arm which was permanently dislocated. [See Appendix 2 for positions to avoid dislocation of the shoulder] Whilst he couldn't feel the arm he could feel acute pain in his shoulder. When receiving personal care the pain became unbearable so he would lash out or grab the offending carer's arm, often bruising them. The hospital tried various splints and pain reducing patches to no avail. Finally, I think the medics just gave up and prescribed unlimited paracetamol. This of course gave him constipation and more pain. Generally, he refused to take the laxatives. He always asked what each of the medications was for.

Finally, about a year before he died a nurse friend of ours who worked at St George's said that paracetamol wasn't appropriate for neurological pain and suggested Pregabelin. This was prescribed immediately and, hooray, it helped no end. Why did it take nine years?

More Issues

For my own sanity I had to sell our car and purchase a vehicle suitable for taking a wheelchair. We didn't qualify for Motability as Murray had his stroke after he was 65. How ageist is that?! It's all to do with the Disability Living Allowance which he wasn't entitled to as he was in receipt of a state pension by then.

In the last three years Murray was entitled to Continuing Healthcare funding. We had a knowledgeable and sympathetic social worker. But he wasn't around for long so when it came to the annual review the next social worker wasn't much help. Thankfully by then a social worker friend who we had known at work came alongside us as our advocate and helped prepare our case for the next couple of years.

Ironically a review was due at about the time Murray died in August 2018. I received a call from the relevant department a few weeks later to invite me to the next meeting to review the funding. They had no idea he had died. To whom had they been paying the money for his care for the last two months? Had the care home not told them he had died? The person concerned got an earful from me.

INS Cares for the Carer

During all this time since I've known about INS, I've been able to ask for help for myself. I was given counselling which helped me to cope with the pressures. No limit on how many sessions. No pressure to get myself right in six sessions! Attended courses such as Taking Back Control. Been part of a Carers' Support group meeting monthly when we share concerns and issues. Felt able to ask advice about financial concerns and entitlements. Have become part of the Spirituality (now Mind, Body, and Spirit) group and shared insights into each other's faith groups. I've had the opportunity to speak to medical students on several occasions about my experiences of being a carer and the help and support I've had from INS.

Amongst all the help we've had from INS one of the greatest things has been the continuity of staff. Even when changes happened the new staff have taken time to get to know the history of their patient. Perhaps this is because it's not a huge unwieldy organisation. INS needs to find a way to get better known in the community, especially amongst the GP practices, community social workers, OTs and care homes.

I had thought that information might be given out with the discharge package from hospital BUT - not such a good idea. There's too much paperwork to handle at that time. It needs to be a little later. Perhaps with a follow up phone call from the social worker on the case at the time of discharge ..... if they haven't already been moved on elsewhere!

~~~~~

Hugh Fells – Carer for Sheila Fells – Stroke Client

Time of Diagnosis

Sheila suffered her stroke when the curtain came down whilst attending the opera "La Bohème" at the Theatre Royal Windsor, during an afternoon performance. We were immediately aware of the situation because of her family history and her various problems with hypertension. On our way up to our friend's house in High Wycombe for lunch prior to our attending the theatre, Sheila was showing signs of being a bit "up tight" whilst in the car. I had recognised this situation for some time and her doctor was in the process of treating her for high blood pressure, commencing with a course of water tablets. She was due to move to a blood pressure tablet regime.

She was removed from the theatre to Wexham Park (South West Bucks Regional Hospital) intensive care unit following a call to para-medics and she was assessed and scanned on arrival. Her immediate family were advised of the situation. Sheila was in intensive care for about five days, following which she was moved to an intermediate ward prior to being transferred to Kingston Hospital. Sheila was diagnosed with a serious bleed on the brain which gave some concern medically at the time, leaving her with left side partial paralysis. Her treatment at Wexham Hospital was very good and we were kept closely advised as to her condition and progress during her stay.

Journey

Sheila was in Kingston Hospital for a number of weeks before being transferred to Putney Hospital in South West London for rehabilitation. Putney was an old hospital and was due for demolition, it was being used mainly for the elderly with one ward for rehab (10 beds). Since not all the
~~~~~

rehab beds were occupied, the elderly inmates were often moved in because of shortages elsewhere, which was distressing for the Rehab group since many of the elderly were end of life cases.

On one occasion Sheila fell whilst trying to leave her bed to attend the toilet, she had been trying to attract the attention of the night staff but without success. We took this up with the administration and asked for a meeting. The impression we got was that the night staff, (one in particular) who were primarily agency employed, were leading busy lives during the day and were not fully awake during the night.

The big help at Putney was the team of New Zealand physiotherapists who really knew their business and put Sheila through her paces, they had her standing and walking (with a stick) in what seemed like a very short time. After leaving Putney Sheila improved through her contacts with organisations working outside the NHS (in particular INS-more later).

After two years, if it were not for her stiff left arm and the use of the walking stick it would have been difficult to detect she had had a stroke at all, her speech and swallowing had returned, and we were able to do most of the things we had previously. She did of course require the use of a wheelchair for longer periods away from the house. A custom-made outdoor version was provided at no cost to us which lasted, with regular servicing, for most of her active life.

Second Stroke

Unfortunately, Sheila suffered a second stroke during the night, an embolism, ten years after her first, on this occasion she was over-weight which did not help the situation, we believe this was largely brought about by her love of good food and being more dependent on her wheelchair, and we her carers had taken our eye off the ball.

We were not altogether happy about the time taken to get her into hospital from the house. It appeared to be a relatively quiet night and the first call was made by a single paramedic who had to await the arrival of the ambulance team which again took some time. She had to be moved down two flights of stairs and finally into the ambulance. The ambulance remained outside for some time before setting off for Kingston Hospital. I do not wish to criticise these operations because I was not fully aware of the medical implications but the wait did seem a long time.

Poor Start to Rehabilitation

Following a period at Kingston Hospital Sheila was moved to Tolworth Hospital for rehabilitation. Following Sheila's rehab and on the day I collected her I noticed a difference in her demeanour, a difference from the evening before and having given it some thought, concluded she had had a TIA (Transient Ischaemic Attack or "mini stroke"), possibly brought about by an anticipation of leaving the hospital and coming home. The staff did not agree. There were no in-house medical staff at Tolworth and when required they had to be called in.

She did not recover an ability to walk, nor talk or swallow and her return home required considerable structural alterations to the ground floor to accommodate her. For all that we took up the challenge and made the most of it and were able to provide a reasonable level of structure to her life. She also had a granddaughter to dote on. Sheila passed away in October of 2018.

Involvement with INS

Following Sheila's return home after the first stroke in July of 1998 we were given a number of leads with regard to extra hospital activities. One was an exercise class in the gymnastic suite which was part of the Richmond Baths complex and run by Different Strokes, an organisation catering for younger stroke sufferers. It was here we met up with the Hughes family who first mentioned the existence of INS, at that time operating from the Kew Baptist Church. INS engaged, in addition to stroke victims, those with Parkinson's and multiple sclerosis (MS). INS grew substantially and moved to a building in Twickenham.

In later years, because of pressure on space and a need to provide for younger clients with neurological problems a number of older clients, Sheila included, moved by agreement to a first-class day centre (Homelink), also in Twickenham.

Sheila enjoyed her time at INS, the morning sessions in Kew and the afternoon communication sessions in Twickenham. During the Kew years every effort was made to arrange outings to various places of interest including the annual Art in Action in Oxford. Sheila joined INS in the autumn of 1998, our association with it has continued for over twenty years.

One very good undertaking was the meetings arranged between doctors and other members of the medical fraternity and INS clients and their carers with the aim of providing a clearer understanding of the needs of people with neurological problems. [See INS work with St George's medical students p173] At the time there was no doubt that members of the non-specialist medical profession sadly lacked a reasonable knowledge of this situation through no fault of their own – they are and were busy people.

INS is very effective as an organisation as is witnessed by its expansion over the years. There is no doubt that after all this time the charity has established a benchmark for excellence in neurological care. If it were a business, it would establish a brand and expand. Other areas of the UK would love to benefit from a professional organisation such as this.

Other Important Factors

Without doubt the opportunity to lead a life which is as normal as can be expected given the existing circumstances. We had spent money on two very important things, both necessary to make life easier, a bed-sit on the ground floor which already had a shower/toilet and utility/kitchen. Because there was a step up to the front door we built a concrete ramp into the garage from the hall and used this as entrance/exit to/from the house. The car's front passenger seat was adapted to swivel outwards allowing easier access. Clearly all this was fine but worth little if the carer was not fit enough to do the man-handling. We counted our blessings I remained fit throughout her ordeal.

We visited Kew Gardens on a regular basis as Friends, Wisley, the Barn near Poole Harbour for a week in Spring with our family and the Hughes family, who also had a disabled member due to a stroke, the seaside town of Porthcawl in Wales and latterly Ross on Wye for a week in the autumn, again with our family and the Hughes. As a group we spent a couple of days each year on the Thames aboard the vessels operated by the charity River Thames Boat Project which is based in Kingston/Teddington.

After Sheila's first stroke we had more flexibility and travelled to Southern Spain, Portugal and Madeira and took three cruises. We watch films at Watermans in Brentford and plays at the Orange Tree and Rose theatres and visited a number of National Trust houses. There was little we could not do, particularly during the first ten years of Sheila's disability we give thanks for that.

~~~~~
~~~~~

Maggie Hughes – Carer for Trevor Hughes – Stroke Client

Time of Diagnosis

Trevor was taken to A&E with a headache, slurred speech and coordination problems which kept coming and going but he was still able to walk, e.g. to the loo. After various tests and X-rays, he was moved to another hospital for a scan where his condition became worse. He was returned to the hospital by which time he appeared to be in pain and unable to walk or speak. It was three weeks before we got a diagnosis.

When the consultant told us he'd had a stroke her manner was very matter-of-fact; that he wouldn't be able to come home from hospital and that I should tell our daughter she wouldn't be able to have a conversation with him (she was eight at the time!). She then turned to the nurse and said something to the effect *"Can you take over here as I have to go and see the 'such and such' family"*. As she left the room I remember saying *"She may be giving up on him but we're not!"* I remember the nurse was kind and sympathetic and aware of the insensitivity of the doctor.

The Journey

Since then, for me and my family, has been long and challenging. Little did we realise on that fateful day 26 years ago that our lives would be changed forever. Trevor, a normally fit and healthy 54-year-old was suddenly unable to walk, read or write or speak intelligibly. We were all in a state of shock. I suddenly found myself thrown into the world of disability trying to manage my work, home and family whilst I was needed at the hospital every day for meetings with the medics and therapists and to interpret Trevor's needs.

My eldest daughter, Lotte who had got married the previous year found out that day that she was expecting their first child. My daughter Alice was working in Italy at the time and was deeply upset and wanted to come home straight away to help. The youngest, Polly was at the local primary school. All three of them have been deeply affected over the years. All the grandchildren were born after Trevor had the stroke so have only known him to be in a wheelchair and unable to hold a 'normal' conversation.

Trevor was to spend almost two years in hospital. Five months in the medical unit at Kingston before being transferred to the Royal Hospital for

Neuro-disability on West Hill, Putney. I organised radical alterations to the house to make his return home possible.

We had to re-think our lives and all our plans for the future as so much would now no longer be possible.

When he left hospital, we were led to believe there was going to be this wonderful team of people all working together to help us. I remember attending a meeting of a group of medics and therapists who were getting together to form this team. Needless to say, none of this materialised and I heard some time later that the team had disbanded due to lack of funding.

He had been offered sessions at a Day Centre for physiotherapy and activities. This was not a success. The one-to-one session soon became a shared group of four patients with one physio whose hours had been reduced and then stopped. There was nothing else suitable there for Trevor and such an air of lethargy about the place that he refused to go. I heard later it had closed.

Somehow over the years we managed to make a life for ourselves through the support of family and friends. Art, music and the creative arts played a large part in this as did our meeting and subsequent friendship with Ellie Kinnear and Liz Grove.

Involvement with INS

I first heard about Ellie from a contact connected with Vineyard Project where I worked as the Art Therapist and deputy organiser. She had Parkinson's and told me she had been greatly helped by a physiotherapist who was setting up a group to help people with neurological conditions using an approach called Conductive Education. She recommended that I contact her for help with Trevor when he came home from hospital.

When we first met Ellie she was running a small group for stroke patients in the lounge of a care home in Twickenham under the guidance of Judit Szathmary, a Conductor trained at the Peto Institute for Conductive Education in Budapest, Hungary.

Ellie was joined by Liz, an occupational therapist (OT) with extensive experience of neurological patients, and other volunteers. Having been told that he would never be able to walk after leaving hospital Ellie and Judit set about changing that way of thinking. Through Judit's Conductive Education programme she encouraged him to use his paralysed side, to stand and walk using a ladder chair, eventually leading him to walking with a narrow-based quad stick and close supervision. [See Appendix 3 for illustration of a ladder chair] He was a good student and worked very hard to improve his situation despite the frustration and limitations of his life. The Stroke group moved into Kew Baptist Church. It was now called 'Holistic Neurological Services".

We met there for several years. Trevor was in the Stroke group of 6-8 people. I joined the Carers group run by Liz and Janette Pye, the social worker. (We still meet after all these years for healthy walks once a month!)

I also started to teach the group art and pottery after the morning sessions with my artist friends Sylvia Des Fours and Bridget Boulting. We involved the INS group in Art and Soul, a charity of which I was a co-founder. We held workshops and exhibitions at Orleans House Gallery. The first time we exhibited INS paintings one was bought by the Henry Boxer Gallery. A joyful moment for one Art Group member, seeing her painting honoured in this way which she had painted with her left hand being unable to use the right hand that she would have normally used.

Our friend Jan came to play the piano and run a Music group with Liz and also Sue Shorter with her percussion instruments.

Trevor made such good progress through Ellie's and Judit's programme involving sitting, standing, lying and walking and Liz's OT support and advice. They always came up with a solution no matter what the problem was.

There were setbacks from time to time. He was knocked over by an automatic door at a respite centre and it took six months rehabilitation to recover from a broken femur.

In 2008 he was diagnosed with cancer and a few days before he was due to go into hospital for a major operation he sang in a concert at St Anne's Church on Kew Green to raise funds for INS. We had a successful exhibition of paintings from the Art group at the Orleans House Gallery at the same time.

'Holistic Neurological Services' became very successful and was renamed Integrated Neurological Services, becoming a charity in 1999. Then it moved to new premises in Hampton Road, Twickenham. Needless to say the waiting list grew with so many more people needing help after experiencing stroke, Parkinson's and other neurological conditions.

In 2011 INS formed a partnership with Homelink Daycare Centre to have a neuro-specific day respite service. This was to be a Tuesday when

INS Physiotherapy, OT and Speech Therapy and Social Work support would be provided at the day respite centre.

Trevor's Stroke group was moved to Homelink which he found quite difficult at first moving to a busy day centre from the intimacy of the small group at INS. Also, the therapy was to cover the needs of many different clients apart from those with stroke. He eventually settled in especially as some of the older members of the group had moved with him and he knew the therapists.

The INS partnership with Homelink came to an end in 2016. In 2016 Trevor had another stroke and I, myself, was unwell with osteoporosis causing me to be less able to give Trevor much physical support. Trevor carried on attending the centre until Covid and lockdowns affected us all.

Homelink have continued to give telephone support and a member of staff comes to spend two hours a week with Trevor for exercise and occupational therapy. INS support has always been offered to us. I belong to the Carers Walking group and to the Mind, Body, and Spirit group with Ellie and Sara Challice. Carol Williams contacts me regularly and keeps us updated on what is going on at INS and in the community.

Trevor and I are still involved with INS after 24 years. We felt very included and well supported as a family. INS is a real lifeline for us.

What Else Has Helped

We have been very fortunate to have Abe, Trevor's Carer/PA who has been helping me to look after him since he first came out of hospital. He understands him so well and we are very lucky to have such dedicated care over such a long period of time. I certainly couldn't have managed without him.

With my involvement in the art world and Trevor's in music our friends and family have all helped to find stimulating things for Trevor to do. Jan from Trevor's Opera group still comes to play the piano for singing sessions. Our sculptor friend, Ralph taught him for many years to paint in his studio whilst listening to Bach. Another artist friend Kate now comes each month to paint with him.

Other organisations that have helped us:

'Share Music' a charity run by Dr Michael Swallow, a retired neurologist and passionate musician. We spent a week in Wales every summer for 10 years with this wonderful organisation working with disabled musicians.

Ottaker Kraus music therapy

Richmond Boat Project - many trips on the river with INS

Companion Cycling - many years of healthy exercise and fresh air in Bushy Park.

The Barn at Holton Lee - memorable breaks at this wonderful nature reserve.

Different Strokes - exercise programme for younger stroke patients where we met Hugh and Sheila Fells whom I referred to INS. Sheila and Trevor were in the same Stroke group and Hugh and I joined the Carers group. We became good friends spending much of our time visiting art galleries, exhibitions, theatres, films and holidays in Dorset and Wales.

~~~~~

Julie Burgess – Carer for Alan Burgess – Stroke Client

Roughly 11.00 p.m. Alan collapsed in the bathroom. When I found him he was unable to get himself up. Alan remembers collapsing and wondering why he could not move his left arm and leg.

Paramedics suspected a stroke when they saw him. We were taken to Charing Cross Hospital. Alan did not lose consciousness. At the hospital they did a CT scan and discovered that Alan had suffered a stroke due to a blood clot in his neck. My first thought was "how do I tell our daughters"?

The following day we were informed that Alan had also lost the sight on the left side of both eyes. It took Alan a while to accept that he had had a stroke. For myself it was like a dream, as though it was happening to someone else.

Alan had to have a cranioplasty two days later as his brain was swelling. Thankfully, the operation worked, and Alan does not seem to remember the days between having the stroke and the op.

As Alan was on the stroke ward it was good to be able to talk to other people about their experiences. Alan had physio in the hospital at least three time a week – I feel that it should have been each day but I know that there are too many patients calling on too few staff.

It was a strange time for both of us. We had to learn new routines and new ways of doing things.
~~~~~

When Alan came home he had a hospital bed downstairs and I used to sleep on a zed bed to be with him. He had community physio which helped greatly. We had carers for the first four weeks and then I took over his care.

How INS Helps

Whilst in the hospital the social worker told us about INS and said that they may be able to help us through things. I referred Alan myself after a few months. I contacted INS but at the time Alan was still too weak to attend the Exercise group on offer. After a few months, when he was stronger, he started at INS one day a week.

At INS he received exercises to suit his needs and the companionship of people who had also been through a stroke. INS are the ones that got Alan back up and walking. Being under INS made us feel that we were not alone, and, in fact, we were doing better than some others.

I have formed many friendships through the INS carers meetings and have been helped immensely by other carers.

We have been with INS for about 11 years and I wish that other sufferers around the country were able to have a service such as INS offer. Presently we are enjoying the INS craft group.

~~~~~

Cia Van der Sluis – Carer for Nigel Vickers-Pocock – Traumatic Brain Injury

Nigel was involved in a road traffic accident while in Greece on holiday. He sustained serious head injury and was transferred to an ICU in Athens where he remained in a coma for five weeks. Awaiting his repatriation to UK, I consulted our GP who strongly advised that on our return, Nigel should be immediately referred to a major teaching hospital specialising in brain injury.

On return by Air Ambulance, despite my best efforts to persuade officials of the urgency for Nigel to be admitted to St George's Hospital, he was admitted to Epsom General Hospital. There a neurologist informed me bluntly that Nigel *"will never change or improve and I should put him in a home"*. I was shocked and asked him the medical basis for this prognosis and his answer was, *"25 years' experience"*.
~~~~~

It soon became clear that Nigel was in the wrong kind of hospital; he needed to be transferred to a specialised environment.

Move to Neurological Hospital – Makes Progress

Although the neurologist was unnecessarily brutal, he did recommend Nigel to The Royal Hospital of Neuro-disability in Putney. Here, now emerged from coma, Nigel's progress was little short of miraculous. He was self-supporting, learning to use a transfer board and with such determination attempting to stand. He was soon seen as a candidate for rehabilitation. Consequently, he was transferred to a neurological rehabilitation centre.

Rehabilitation – Setbacks

At the centre there was no resident doctor. Care was provided by a variety of therapists, nurses and care assistants. Soon, a programme of drugs was prescribed and administered to Nigel, without my knowledge. Immediately his condition deteriorated being marked by: increasing desire to sleep; decreasing ability to concentrate; and, no longer having the ability to self-support.

I contacted three individual neurologists who got back to me with the same opinion, that he should not be on this mixture or amount of drugs. The Trust's own neurologist actually said they would do Nigel "more harm than good".

After a long battle regarding the medication, he was transferred to a hospital particularly involved in care for people with disabling head injuries, in order to have the drugs reduced. On changing his anti-convulsant, which I strongly objected to, he suffered further physical disability to his left side.

There is a Better Way

Clearly, serious head injury demands specialist medical attention from the very first day. It requires a wide range of neurological consultants and therapists to prescribe and carry out appropriate treatment. It was Nigel's right to expect and receive this quality of care. Sadly, he was denied it.

The officials arranging his transfer from Gatwick Airport completely ignored my well-informed pleas and despatched him to Epsom General Hospital which was ill-equipped to receive such a patient and the procedures fell far short of being able to provide a reliable first opinion.

The infamous death or cabbage prognosis was informally passed, and the current view would have had Nigel consigned to the negative, inactive environment of a residential nursing home. It would also have denied Nigel the opportunity of showing what he could do, free of the offending neuroleptic drugs.

Had there been one professional body from the first day, to diagnose, advise, monitor, provide the mental and physical therapies required and see the patient and family all the way through their journey, I have no doubt it would have played a crucial, beneficial and financial part in saving, not only the family, but the whole of the NHS an incredible amount of time and money.

In summary: Nigel came home having two carers, 24/7, 365 days a year. This could have been avoided, at the very least, halved, had he been in an appropriate hospital or under a professional team, given the correct diagnosis and rehabilitated to the best he could have been.

How INS Supports and Improves the Client's Daily Life

Nigel's profession was a surveyor but his love in life was singing which he did with a pianist in various venues. I happened to see an INS poster advertising a concert in Kew. I had never heard of INS but thought it might be something Nigel would enjoy. It was a wonderful concert. After the concert I met Ellie Kinnear founder of INS who explained who they were. That was the beginning of a long relationship with INS to this day.

Now at home, I had to search on my own for various outlets for Nigel. There was no one-body in our area that could provide any help or advice for people severely handicapped with neurological conditions.

INS provides therapies, classes, outings and get-togethers for their clients. Although we were based in a different borough, INS allowed us to make use of their facilities. Ellie Kinnear introduced us to a music therapy teacher, Margaret Lobo, the founder of the Otaker Kraus Music Trust, where Nigel attended on a regular basis and loved.

Another very important issue that INS were able to help us with was physiotherapy. Ellie Kinnear came to our home to teach myself and the statutory carers how to assist Nigel in stretching his limbs prior to washing and dressing him, the importance of correct seating and the normality of posture.

A while after Nigel passed away in 2017, I was fortunate to be able to volunteer at INS where I assisted in the Art group up until the Covid Lockdown.

I am only sorry that services such as INS cannot be rolled out to all parts of the country. This sort of organisation is rare but there is a real demand. Accidents and neurological conditions happen to so many people and yet the Authorities fail to provide little, if any, help or assistance for those starting out on an horrific and very lonely journey.

As so many Rehabilitation centres have closed, we need now more than ever, organisations to step in from day one to advise, guide and support the clients and their families through an extremely emotional and complex road ahead. This should be continued until the client has reached their full potential.

~~~~~

Sara Challice – Carer for Neal Challice – Brain Tumour Client

Very Difficult Times – Before and After Diagnosis

Neal was misdiagnosed for many months before he was finally diagnosed with a brain tumour. His GP prescribed him cranial relaxants, but when I enquired on how Neal felt and if they were helping – they did not. He just felt woozy, but the side-effects of the tumour remained. It wasn't until Neal couldn't stand up anymore, that I called for an ambulance. After a night in A&E, and a few bags of saline on a drip (Neal was unable to eat or drink due to the pressure of the tumour in his head), they sent him home with a couple of paracetamol. I did question the doctor at the time and asked, "Is that it?!"

It seemed very odd. Twenty-four hours later, I had to admit Neal into hospital again, as he was back to being unable to stand, drink or eat. The A&E staff looked surprised, and I refused to allow him home until they gave him further tests. He was kept in overnight on the observatory ward, had an MRI scan the next day, and then diagnosed with a brain tumour.

As Neal was in West Middlesex hospital, there was little they could do. He needed to be admitted to Charing Cross hospital for an operation. I called Charing Cross hospital and spoke to the sister on the ward. She was abrupt and rude, saying that even if Neal was admitted to her ward that
~~~~~

day, they wouldn't operate for a week. I continued to press her and she hung up on me. I knew Neal had very limited time. As I made my way back to Neal's hospital ward, despondent, staff made us aware that an ambulance was on its way and the sister at Charing Cross hospital had organised for Neal to come in and be admitted to the last bed available in her ward. She was rude upon arrival! But we didn't care – Neal's life was hanging in the balance and he was where he needed to be! He was operated on within the week.

My Involvement with INS

I have been involved with INS for over 10 years. Once I knew INS were rebranding and had a new logo, I said to not spend any more money on design agencies and that I would help design their collateral, and produce leaflets, newsletters, posters, and digital marketing. This is when I was asked to be a Trustee for the charity, for which I was for five years – as both a carer representative and as the designer of their marketing materials.

After my husband passed, I decided I needed a break and stood down as a Trustee, but continued to take the Mind, Body, and Spirit group with Ellie Kinnear once a fortnight, for both clients with neurological conditions and carers.

A Better Way Forward

I remember at one INS AGM, an elderly gentleman in a wheelchair, disabled after having a stroke, sharing his story:

"When I was diagnosed and sent home from hospital, I sat in my wheelchair, gazing out of the back window and I thought that this was it, my life was over – but INS has shown me that this there is so much more!"

INS views a client beyond their disablement and supports each individual, mentally, emotionally, and physically. INS give a holistic approach – empowering those diagnosed to help look after themselves and to stay well for as long as possible. This not only gives clients a better quality of life but can even extend their lives. This also helps to lower admissions to hospital, saving our economy money.

INS is invaluable and very much needed as we become an ageing population, with more of us needing neurological support and help within the community. INS is truly unique and I feel needs to be rolled out at a national level.

Important Lessons

I never gave up hope for Neal and would leave no stone unturned! After Neal had a stroke and was unable to speak, I took him to a homeopath in St Margaret's – Dr Innes. This doctor had been a general practitioner and then fallen very ill himself. Pharmaceutical drugs were not helping and he finally put an advert in the back of a medical journal asking for help. The replies led him to nutrition, homeopathy, and herbalism – complementary medicine – which helped to heal him, and he now works as a homeopath and herbalist.

Neal was prescribed a simple supplement – Cytozyme-B, which is condensed lambs' brain. After six weeks of taking this, it was like Neal "woke up". He was suddenly able to speak and turn his head again. It was a revelation! Something had clearly healed in his brain, and I could only put it down to this supplement.

Unfortunately, nutrition is rarely considered by doctors and healthcare specialists. For the 13 years Neal was ill from a brain tumour, his doctors never mentioned that sugar promotes cancer growth. I now know much more when it comes to our diet – and we need to help support our bodies with organic fruit and vegetables, as well as having 6-8 glasses of water a day. This will help support those with neurological conditions – to empower them to improve their diet, giving them more energy and to support their health.

~~~~~
~~~~~

Chapter 3
Real-Life Experience – Parkinson's, MS

CLIENTS

Bindu Thakrar – PD Client

The Start of My Journey

In late 2009 my left leg was shaking involuntarily even when I sat at my desk at work. I was a Project Manager in the IT department of a large retail bank. I was referred to a private neurologist who did some blood tests and an X-ray and MRI scan but he did not give a diagnosis. I had a bereavement - my brother passed away in May 2010 - and so my diagnosis was put on hold.

I went to my mum's house for 14 days to pay respects to my brother and had prayers in the evenings and attended the funeral aware of my tremor. My mum thought that the tremor was due to my feeling cold and shock from the tragedy that had hit us all very hard. Then at the end of June my father-in-law became unwell so again my condition went unattended, and all our attention was on him and his recovery.

In July I was finally able to focus on myself. In August 2010 at the next appointment with my neurologist I was accompanied by my daughter. The neurologist booked an appointment for me to have a Datscan, an X-ray of the brain, and that was when I was told that I had Parkinson's. He put me on a course of medication - Sinemet. At that time, I had no idea what Parkinson's was but was relieved we had reached a diagnosis.

During all of this I was still grieving for the loss of my brother and the worry of my father-in-law's health as well as doing my job and caring for my husband and two daughters.

The next worry was how I was going to be treated. As I hadn't seen or met anyone with Parkinson's before I felt very anxious about the tremors and felt very lonely as I wasn't sure what was going on and how I would be affected by it. My husband tried to calm me by doing research on the Internet because when I tried I was just getting more worried and panicky which didn't help.

My husband and daughters were trying their best to keep my spirits up. At this stage I hadn't told my mum or any of my family but I knew I would have to soon.

When my GP referred me to a different neurologist at the National Hospital for Neurology and Neurosurgery in Queen Square, Holborn, the neurologist there advised me that the medication I was on was not the best for me as I had just been diagnosed and should be on a much lower dosage of a lesser strength medication to start with and increase dosage/strength as and when required in the future.

Whilst all this was going on I was unable to give 100% to my job so I was put on sick leave and then in 2011 my husband suggested I leave my job as the commute was very long and stressful.

Involvement with INS

My GP referred me to the Parkinson's Rehab team at Heart of Hounslow which ran a course for newly diagnosed Parkinson's patients in March 2012. It was run by the Parkinson's nurse and it was at this course that I learned of INS from one of the other attendees and what services they provided.

When I got in touch with INS they advised me that I could do a self-referral which I did in November 2012. Since then, I have been attending the courses and group activities they run throughout the year for nine years.

INS was just what I needed as we were a group of clients in the same boat although at different stages, different symptoms and different medications. The group forum allowed for all of us to share experiences which gave me a lot of information and insight of what was to come and how I may be affected by Parkinson's going forward.

The main PD group session was run fortnightly by a physio where we discussed any changes to our health, changes to medications etc. and exchanged information that would be of interest to others such as dance classes, craft sessions as well as community events etc. We also had an exercise session using gym equipment which focused on the relevant aspects of keeping balance and mobility. During these sessions we also learned about Nordic walking using poles.

INS also offered other courses such as sleep management, speech and language therapy, counselling, creative writing, art, music sessions, mind body spirit, and also mindfulness, to name a few. All of these are run by qualified professional staff.

INS also organises sessions for medical students from St George's Medical School to talk to clients with neurological disorders which I volunteer to attend.

The groups which have especially helped me are sleep management, speech and language therapy, mind, body, and spirit, and the exercise session, which all include time to discuss problems with an opportunity to share information and advice. The Mind, Body, and Spirit group has been very calming, and we discuss various books such as those of Anita Moorjani, Eckhart Tolle, and articles, and everyone makes very useful contributions.

What Else Has Helped

Through INS I have gained a lot of knowledge about my condition and been supported by professional qualified people in a friendly and caring way. Also very helpful is sharing experiences with others in the same boat and making friends that can relate to my issues and my feelings and be very supportive in ways that family and friends aren't always able to.

~~~~~

Bharti Patel – PD Client

Time of Diagnosis

I was given the diagnosis of Parkinson's in July 2008. The GP referred me to the neurology consultant, Dr Pearce, who still sees me now at Charing Cross Hospital instead of West Middlesex. My husband was present at the first meeting with Dr Pearce when he gave me the diagnosis. There was little to no support for my husband or children – a son and a daughter. It was a shock to them. They were a bit upset. The symptoms started with tremor in the left hand and dragging of the left foot. I was given only medication.

The Journey

There was no support for the family and no physical support was offered to me.

I used to work in Barclays Bank. I took early retirement in 2013 aged 59
~~~~~

Involvement with INS

I saw an INS poster in the Teddington office of the NHS Benefits department in 2012. I referred myself. An INS physiotherapist saw me at home first and then I joined a Parkinson's group, which I enjoyed. Another physiotherapist took me Nordic Walking and I also did hydrotherapy in the Teddington Pool.

I was thrilled to be offered water skiing with the INS Expanding Horizons Programme and found that I was successful, much to my family's surprise. I attended by the R70 bus or my husband brought me. I am still involved with INS taking part in a Zoom Parkinson's group programme run by a physiotherapist.

If I get emotional then my tremor increases, but when I took the Mindfulness Meditation group I felt much calmer. I now practise this on my own. I find the staff friendly, and I feel safe.

What Else Has Helped

I also do regular yoga since 1990. I joined a Parkinson's Dance Class in 2012 which stopped in 2015. Now I take part in a Ballet Dance group for people with PD in Kingston run by an ex-ballerina and her husband. I like walking in nature watching the birds.

Making the Service More Effective

Increase the services. I would like to have been referred to INS at the time of diagnosis.

~~~~~

Jon McPherson – PD Client

A Tough Time

In 1995 I fell from a helicopter while abseiling at 200 feet. It felt as if the rope had been pulled from my hand. I fell fully kitted about 150 feet in two seconds, I only had 30 feet to go when a safety man on the ground managed to recover the rope and Save My Life, a hard pill to swallow. As I believe, I should be dead, no question.

My wife was always aware that family come second to any soldier; the army comes first. During our marriage I spent six months in Bosnia, eight months in the Glasshouse, Colchester military correction centre, two months in Canada and many weeks away training. Perhaps in total I must
~~~~~

have spent two to three years away from my family. We left the forces in 2001

Another Tough Journey

I became unwell in 2009 and continued to work for two years. My symptoms were unknown or in other words my GP didn't have a clue. Her advice when I asked could it be Parkinson's was "go away get yourself fit stop being so ridiculous I don't want to see you for another three months".

So, I took the advice of my GP and spent the next 18 months trying to find out what was wrong with me. I spent thousands of pounds, was medicated through Combat Stress for PTSD and severe Chronic Anxiety then was sent to Vanbrugh Hill Clinic in Greenwich.

The GP took one look at me before I could sit down said "you've got Parkinson's". As I sat down I said "how do you know", he said "it's obvious and I can't believe you've not been diagnosed yet". He then referred me for a brain DAT scan. I was then informed by Professor Pacini at Charing Cross hospital that it was Parkinson's and I had it for at least two years.

I then said "thanks very much" stood up to walk out and my wife said "well you took that very well" to which I replied "now I'm going to be properly medicated, no more of that pregabalin". I did hope to get better and get back into work, but it never works out that way unfortunately.

Symptom after symptom starts to creep in and then as luck would have it I was referred to INS. I also was being treated for PTSD and Chronic Anxiety, INS agreed to deal with the mental and physical side and had me working with the groups.

INS for me was a life saver, 47 counselling sessions, group meetings and I teach Creative Writing. INS is a great charity that has supported me through this illness and so I want to raise as much money as possible to go towards its vital work! Without INS, I really don't know where I would be.

How to Climb a Mountain

I raised money climbing Bennachie, a range of hills in Aberdeenshire with several tops, the highest of which, Oxen Craig, has a height of 528m (1733 feet).

This was an amazing challenge. For me Parkinson's is totally unpredictable, meaning I suddenly freeze, movements are slow, horrendous back pain, tremor, I basically have no control and at times through the day, I cannot stand, walk, or even keep my balance.

The climb started at 9am in the morning. The experience was at first one of increased anxiety, stress and doubt, knowing in my mind that I was more than capable of achieving this goal but in reality, I had no idea whether I was going to be physically and mentally able to do the walk.

There was no way I could have completed the task on my own, my symptoms are so unpredictable and can leave me exhausted before I have even started....so, I decided I could only achieve this with my long-time friend and colleague from the Army Air Corps, Warrant Officer II Stephen Fisher and another friend outside of the army, Pete Bakker.

With the military mind set, there had to be no ifs and buts, no doubts, the challenge was there, and it had to be achieved. INS dragged me out of a very dark place, and without their continued support, I really don't know where I'd be now. The support from INS has helped me to take back control and learn to pace myself. I have been able to swim and cycle in order to create some stamina/ strength when it was needed, which came after about 20 feet into the climb, only 1746 feet to go I thought to myself.

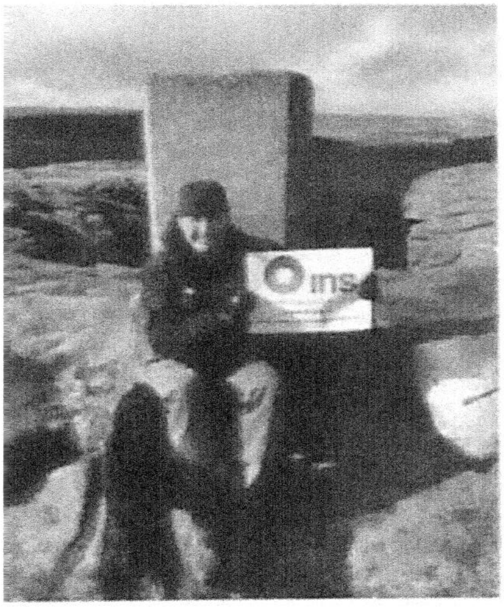

Once I got a pace going and made use of the Nordic sticks (taught by INS) my walking was pretty good. Each time I stopped for a minute or two, then freezing mode sets in and suddenly I've forgotten how to walk. There was a moment when I slipped going up, Pete dived on me in a flash, then coming down, Pete slipped and I was on top of him in a flash; it's incredible really, how the disease can control you, yet in order to save someone my brain allowed me to act without thought.

So, the top conquered, and back down to the car, in a record time of 2 hours 45 minutes, set by us. I'm thinking of doing the same again for INS, but it took me over a month to recover, so I need to give it some thought nearer the time. The walk was actually scheduled for the previous day but due to the weather, rain and wind, I'd probably still be up there now!

I think the most daunting part of the 4-day trip to Aberdeen was going through airport security. Every symptom, despite taking my medication, comes out to present you to everyone around you...horrendous, but raising £2,850 for INS was wonderful!

~~~~~

Nick Berners-Price - Living with MS

Nick is Programme Director, 4D Life. www.4dlife.org

I have multiple sclerosis, an auto immune condition that finds the immune system attacking the nervous system for unknown reasons. This process results in demyelination, holes or lesions in the myelin sheath that surrounds and protects nerves. Symptoms can include almost anything, but commonly problems with eyesight, sensation, energy levels, brain fog, bladder control and ultimately movement.

My first symptoms appeared in January 2006, six months after the birth of my eldest son. I woke up with numbness in my feet, which progressed up my legs gradually over the next few months.

My GP initially suspected Guillain-Barre syndrome and referred me to a neurologist. MRI scans showed up nothing, and a wait-and-see approach was adopted. By this stage chronic fatigue had set in, making a flight of stairs quite a challenge. I remember turning over in bed and getting out of breath. I decided that I must find something to make a difference, some kind of solution.

The irony is that I am a personal trainer, my job involving helping people lose weight, get fit and sometimes run marathons and climb mountains. I had been doing this for over 10 years. I was booked in to climb Mount Kilimanjaro that winter!

I had become fascinated by the human body and how it works when I was 14 years old, making a career out of helping people use exercise and nutrition to enhance their lives. I realised I now had to dig much deeper, see if I could find solutions to help my own situation, and maybe others in similar situations.

15 years on and I now work entirely with people with medical conditions, using an approach split into four dimensions – movement, nutrition, function, and lifestyle. There is so much evidence now that
~~~~~

almost all neurological conditions and injuries can be significantly helped through these factors, as well as through medication. Researching and following the evidence has brought me into contact with so many people that have knowledge and experience that can improve lives, reduce symptoms and slow or stop progression. But so often this knowledge and experience is not presented to people living with neurological injury or disease.

And for those who do come across it, the difficulty comes in knowing what to do and how to do it.

15 years ago I radically improved my diet, stopped trying to exercise in a way that made me look good and run faster, starting instead to exercise and shape my lifestyle in a way that made me healthier. After 18 months I was virtually symptom free.

That's not to say I am now. Life has thrown many hurdles and pitfalls in the way of living a perfect lifestyle. And it was confirmed sometime later that I have multiple sclerosis. But I am convinced, and the evidence does much of that convincing, that the way I live my life and my exercise, nutrition and functional training has been central to the fact that I still lead a full and rewarding life 15 years on. The challenges of raising two sons and running two businesses might well have been overwhelming without this.

Whatever you choose to call it – whole body, holistic, integrated, functional - this type of approach is vital to successfully improving outcomes. Life is challenged in so many ways by neurological injury or condition and the solution is to adopt a marginal gains attitude.

Looking for ways to feel better and reduce symptoms in as many areas as possible, no matter how small the gain.

These many marginal gains cumulatively result in feeling significantly better and living well with your condition rather than being diminished by it.

And the psychological element here is perhaps the most important. The right exercise, nutrition, function and lifestyle training lifts your mood, tackles anxiety and depression, creates a positive outlook and a vision for a positive future that allows life to be fully lived.

~~~~~
~~~~~

CARERS

Stuart Banks – Carer for Gail Banks – MS Client

The Initial Shock

Gail was diagnosed in October 1990. Multiple Sclerosis. We had heard of it, but the phrase, "neurological disease" was uncharted territory as far as we were both concerned. I know for certain that at the consultation we both thought imminent death from this condition, so understandably we were in total shock. Death and foreboding, it being the beginning of the end. We didn't speak of our experience of that day until several years after, surprisingly. For two young people who had two young children and everything to look forward to, the phrase "frightened and cheated" comes to mind.

The consultant did mention that it wasn't to be taken as a death sentence as there were ways that they could help. The positive aspect was that it was relapsing remitting MS. However positive that may seem it still didn't register. Counselling was offered together with medication that could alleviate symptoms.

Still, it was that terminology, "neurological" that stuck in both our minds – that's to do with the brain! So many questions that we both wanted to ask but were scared to ask; how will this condition affect Gail physically and mentally? How do we explain to the family, including the children? How will we answer the questions that we don't know the answer to? Gail later confided with her mother asking, how can I do this to Stuart? I can't be the same Gail that he loved and married – how can I go on like this?

On my part, I thought that any thought of my future was selfish and insignificant. From now on, it must be Gail and the children only and not a thought for my well-being. We were somewhat fortunate in some respects, as the hospital that diagnosed Gail's condition happened to be the centre for ARMS – Action and Research into Multiple Sclerosis. Therefore, they had an advantage in treating and advising us on the issues. However, it was 1990 and it wasn't too long before budgetary restrictions negated their ongoing support.

The Horror of Uncertainty

As mentioned, for what seemed an eternity, we remained unsure of exactly what the journey would be. As much as Gail remained positive on the outside, she would often break down in tears, fearing our relationship, will she remain able to be a mum - will she become too disabled to carry on? Her mum once told me that Gail had tried to make her promise that if she became so disabled to the point that she was incontinent or needed care, that she would want to end her life, and would her mum help her? As for my children, they asked is mummy going to die? They had picked up on something, probably the constant visits to the hospital etc. We really regretted that it came to the point when they asked us, but we really weren't sure of the answers...we tried to shield them.

A Turn for the Worse – The Challenges of Coping

Gail carried on with life, working and enjoying our family. Severe fatigue and the occasional fall for the best part of 16 years was the norm. However, August 2006 Gail had a seizure in the early hours. We learned that she had a UTI (urinary tract infection) that hadn't been treated appropriately and that it had festered for a long time. Gail didn't fully recover from that episode. From there on, her condition deteriorated considerably. During her stay in hospital, it became apparent that MS had reared its ugly head to the full.

She became incontinent (double incontinence) could no longer communicate verbally and her physical deterioration was shocking. Gail remained in hospital for three months, mainly in a rehabilitation ward (now closed). Although I was able to learn how to cope to a certain extent with the degree of her disability when she came home, I was ill prepared for most of the challenges that were to come.

From 2006 – 2009 Gail spent many more months in hospital, mainly as a result of UTI's becoming the ruling factor. Various treatments, various specialised units onwards, it was becoming clear that there was a fragmented system that I found almost impossible to navigate. So many hospitals, so many aspects of social care that were not joining up made me feel like giving up...but I couldn't!

Then, at a visit to Gail's consultant at West Middlesex Hospital in 2009, I asked the consultant *"Why am I having to deal with all this, why am I not getting help, why do I feel like I'm constantly arranging and calling so many departments and having to rely on self-help?"* I had admitted to myself, I've had enough, and this is reflecting on Gail's health and well-being. With her head in her hands, she answered *"Stuart, I'm so sorry. The standard of care and after care within the NHS is just not there"*

Although shocked at first, it confirmed that my findings were genuine. She then referred me to INS. By this time however, Gail had become so disabled that she could not engage with many of the areas that INS specialised in.

INS Provides a Better Way Forward with Support for the Carer

However, it's what INS did for me that really helped. As well as regularly assessing Gail at home, they looked closely at what my needs were. They taught me how I could cope better, explained the nature of the condition that Gail had. Everything from physio techniques, speech, and language therapy; a journey that helped me to help Gail and helped me to realise that I have a life.

I had a wonderful outlet from a member of INS. We would meet regularly just to have a coffee and a chat. I was able to let lose my anguish and feel confident that there was a way. Although Gail's condition had worsened and it was too late for total involvement, the help and encouragement I received was so valuable. I was asked to volunteer at the INS MS group. There, I was invited to take part in helping at the physio sessions; after they were satisfied they had taught me the basics. I was thrilled that I could help and in turn, I could help Gail.

A couple of years later I was offered a post at INS and my role in life changed in such a positive way it's hard to put into words. A revelation to me that in turn helped Gail. I was so happy that they had seen things from a different angle entirely.

I have been involved with INS for 12 years – as a volunteer and as a full-time staff member 2013 – 2015. It has worked with a supreme ethos; it has engaged where others have failed to go. It is loved by the clients and carers and offers practical advice, sessions for physio and occupational therapy, outings for clients and carers – emotional and physical support for clients and carers. There is a uniqueness with INS which is in the name. Hope, is for me the main ingredient, backed up with practical and emotional support.

There hasn't been a lot of help outside of INS. The journey includes care company involvement, the Department for Work and Pensions, the NHS and all the problems of everyday living because those issues don't pass over you. That's the Integration aspect; INS largely stands alone with its ethos.

Making the System More Effective

The care system needs to change direction, particularly concerning neurological conditions. Since 2012, I have tried and as yet failed to help defragment the care system by engaging with MP's, NHS consultants, Community Health, etc. My hope is that one day, someone will sit up and listen. Various governments have hailed their intention to integrate the NHS and Social Care. How? I could expand given the time and a platform, but I am assured of one thing; integration needs a model.

The present system is crying out for change and those changes do not mean millions of pounds being thrown into the system. What the system needs is radical change that is measured and open to new ideas that revolutionise the care system.

A system should be targeted specifically, and neurological conditions are an excellent target. We know that the knowledge and understanding of these conditions is at the very least poor at NHS and Social Care levels.

Paid Carers Guided and Supported by a Neuro Team

I feel that the time is now, to look at total care from the time of diagnosis and create a system that takes a neuro team into the homes of clients that need care; specialised, trained home carers. When the family can no longer cope alone there is a need for a Caring Service that addresses the needs of both the patient and the family carer with the guidance of a neurological team. The aim is for the carers to help maintain a person's independence for as long as possible. This can be done by guiding the carers to maintain the client's mobility and strength as part of their daily routine. This will help them support the person more easily and create a positive atmosphere. In the early days after a stroke on discharge home this will allow the client to keep on improving thus requiring the carer to give less physical help and give them a feeling of pride in seeing their client improve. [See p187-188 on the effectiveness of such care support]

There are many aspects, many hurdles but they can be overcome. It will take radical changes. A model of a new integrated care system can be the model for all to follow. Exciting times, let's be brave and invent. It can be done!

~~~~~
~~~~~

Keith Severs – Carer for Pat Severs – PD Client

Initial Diagnosis

Pat started showing signs and experiencing symptoms of PD from the mid-1990s, though we did not recognise them as PD at the time. We shared the common misconception that PD always meant tremor, which Pat never had (about a third of people with PD never have tremor). Pat's early signs were occasional but increasing inability – N.B. inability, not just difficulty - to get up from a chair and regular inability to turn over in bed.

Surprisingly, our GP misdiagnosed Pat's condition as arthritis. In April 1998, some three years after her first PD signs, we stayed with a friend, a pathologist, who suggested Pat should see a neurologist. At Pat's first appointment, the consultant diagnosed PD. Since Pat had no tremor we had guessed she probably had MS. So, Pat must be the only person ever to be relieved to be told she had PD, given she had no idea how bad it could, and eventually did, become. The consultant prescribed Levodopa but offered no advice other than contacting the PD Society.

Shortly afterwards we attended our first Richmond PD Society meeting. Ellie Kinnear was also there, explaining the benefits of INS. So, Pat promptly asked to join.

What Followed – A 13 Year Journey

Ellie came to our home to assess Pat. I took Ellie into the living room and said I would leave them to it. Ellie then forcefully made clear that Pat's PD was as much my concern as Pat's, so I should stay. And of course, she was absolutely right. Ellie spelled out the therapeutic and wider benefits of INS, and my role in helping Pat manage PD. Pat then became an INS client for the rest of her life.

By this time, Pat's failure to turn over in bed had worsened from frequent to constant. She had also begun to experience "freezing", involuntary complete stoppages caused by PD but often stress induced. For instance, the fear of being unable to walk across a pedestrian crossing would prompt the very result she feared, and we'd stand there immobile, enduring the expletives of naturally irate drivers.

From INS we learned the two countermeasures to freezing: concentration and rhythmic movement, in the latter case led by me. Pat found Glen Miller's "In the Mood" worked best for her. This, however, was not to be recommended when in a crowded supermarket. Similar to freezing was hesitation when walking through doorways, especially where a time factor was involved, like entering lifts or tube carriages, where PD effects were accentuated by her fear of being stranded on the other side of the doors from myself. Eventually our use of public transport was limited to buses, where Pat's fear of being left behind was offset by the knowledge that the driver would not shut the door in her face.

Naturally, medication mitigated PD effects. But this was complicated by Pat's drug routine. This initially consisted of two main dosages, Levodopa only, at 7am and 3pm with an overnight top-up at 11pm. Each daytime dose was actually an overdose thereby causing dyskinesias, involuntary violent jerking movements, in her case of the trunk and arms, lasting from seconds to several minutes. The short Levodopa half-life meant dyskinesia was followed by a long period of relative normality then a spell, albeit shorter, of PD effects, all twice daily. This entailed planning our life to minimise activities between about 1pm to 4pm every day.

For the next few years Pat's PD was mainly confined to leg movement and was largely creeping deterioration. My role during this period was mainly helping Pat going to bed, turning her over during the night and getting her up and helping her shower and dress in the morning, and help with walking. It was fortunate that I was physically capable of doing these; had our roles been reversed Pat wouldn't have been able to budge me at all.

Pat at this time was able to move relatively easily about the house, with flat even floors and plenty of objects to grab but walking outdoors was a far more hostile environment. Pat had acquired the notorious Parkinson's shuffle from an early stage causing her to trip over raised paving stones and, as her balance deteriorated, stumble on uneven surfaces. So she always needed someone to accompany her, gripping her arm, when outside home. This role largely fell to me, and Pat called me her gaoler. PD effects varied from day to day, and on good days she managed walking quite well. Pat would then beg me to let go, which I refused to do. But foolishly one day I relented; Pat immediately tripped, fell and cracked her pelvis. (People with PD tend to fall like tree trunks with little or no attempt to break the fall.)

We had always shared household chores, but there was now a gradual increase in my doing these, limited by Pat's own insistence on doing as much as she could manage.

I had carried on working part time but gave that up in 2001, three years after her diagnosis. Pat looked after her medication and its timetable. She also cooked as much as possible, especially when entertaining. We maintained social activities as much as circumstances permitted, but attendance at crowded functions had to be given up from an early stage because of practical problems like getting to the loo through a crowd.

From about 2003 Pat's PD began to spread beyond her legs, with handwriting and speech – both clarity and volume - and manual functioning deteriorating. Pat had always maintained contact with her numerous friends by phone but sadly this had to be first curtailed and then abandoned because her friends could not understand anything she said. On the plus side, a change of PD consultant led to a complete revamp of her drug regime, with the three daily dosages replaced by 10 – yes 10 – and increased use of agonistes and continuous release Levodopa. Dyskinesias vanished overnight.

The listing below shows her daily drug regime in 2011. This stabilised Pat throughout the day but only partly restored her verbal facility. I had then to take full responsibility for administering her drugs because Pat could no longer physically manage them.

But this drug regime presented a problem, one regularly experienced by people with PD, when she had to stay in hospital for three weeks for an unrelated condition. The ward doctor promptly amended – distorted might be a more appropriate word - her drug regime to fit in with the regular three times daily drug delivery. I protested, emphasising the serious effects Pat would suffer; his response was "I'm the doctor here, not you". When I told him I would have to enlist the support of Pat's PD consultant, he backed down and agreed that I could administer her drugs. So, I spent each day, all day, at hospital with her, except for the early morning/late evening doses which the ward nurses agreed to provide.

Eventually, about three years before she died, Pat was on the maximum safe dosage of Agonistes and Amantadine and the choice had to be made between increased immobility or a recurrence of dyskinesias, caused by larger Levodopa dosages; Pat opted for the latter. The dyskinesias, however, were no longer the violent movements previously experienced but a more continuous lower-level activity.

By this time, Pat could no longer fend for herself at all, and even had difficulty reading, spending most of her time watching TV or chatting to visitors. She also had difficulty downing liquids yet could swallow runny food, so soups became the order of the day.

Pat declined the use of a wheelchair until absolutely necessary which was about a year before she died.

INS' Role – Making a Difference

Throughout her long decline Pat received continuous support from INS. Although difficult to quantify, it would be hard to overstate the benefits Pat obtained. The weekly group therapy alone would be enough, but there was so much more: for instance, immediate advice, practical assistance, discussions, play reading sessions, and art classes. There were also group outings such as a trip on the boat Richmond Adventurer on the Thames, visiting Kew Gardens, and companion tandem cycling in Bushey Park, plus the asset of being part of the INS community, with everyone an individual, not just an NHS number.

INS's support provided constant reassurance without which Pat would have floundered and worried considerably, and so was vital for her mental well-being.

So, I feel very strongly that Pat, without INS's help and support, would not have coped with PD as well as she actually managed. This is underlined by the contrast between her progress and that of her sister Joyce, who also had PD. Joyce did not have the good fortune to live in the INS catchment area, so had no therapy and only minimal support; her decline was very much faster than Pat's.

Given constant financial constraints, it is a miracle INS achieves so much. "Neuro-support for life" is INS's motto: and that is exactly what it delivers.

Incidentally, it is a well-known fact that certain substances trigger PD, the chief culprit being agricultural fertiliser. Evidence indicates that there is a possible familial factor determining who acquires PD this way. And it is clear that the trigger is latent, being set in childhood but activated in old age. Pat and her sister were born and bred in Swansea. Pat left Swansea to work in London and Joyce stayed in Swansea till her marriage in her twenties. So why am I mentioning them in this context? Because both were evacuated during the war to farms in west Wales. It was Pat's consultant's belief that their PD trigger was set during this period.

In addition to being Pat's carer, I helped with the organisation and running of fundraising events such as bottle tombolas at Kew, Richmond and Twickenham fairs, Scottish dancing and other themed evenings, ferret races, street collections and the Annual Grand draw, and have continued helping in a similar capacity since Pat died. Both Pat and I were also regular participants in the St George's Medical School students' sessions when students visit INS to learn about its objectives and methods. It also helps them understand the reality from both the patient's and carer's point of view.

My Experience as a Carer

This was much easier for me than for most carers in that:

1. I was physically able to meet the demands of lifting Pat from chairs or bed and helping her to get in and out of cars etc. INS carers' meetings at the time were like Groundhog Day, with female carers repeatedly complaining about backache caused by manhandling their charges.

2. With PD being progressive, my role began as caring light, and I was able to gradually grow into the role and adapt as requirements changed.

3. I had a full private pension and therefore had no major financial problems. Carers in employment might well face severe financial hardship if forced to choose paying for daytime care or giving up work to provide the necessary help themselves.

4. I was in good health. Many PD carers are elderly themselves and are likely to have medical conditions impacting on their caring capability (INS actually had a PD client who was himself the main carer of his wife who had motor neurone disease).

5 As well as our daughters, we had many friends, able and willing to help.

6 And last but not least, I benefited considerably as a carer from my involvement with INS, both from advice and help from the professionals and learning from other carers' experience: invaluable!

Over time, as Pat aged and deteriorated, the time taken by my caring steadily increased eventually becoming 24/7. As Pat's needs increased, so her friends' ability to help waned since her female helpers no longer had the strength to cope. When Pat permanently needed help when using the lavatory, assistance from men friends was ruled out. So, except for our daughters' help, the caring duty fell totally on me. But by then I had become fully accustomed to looking after Pat on a daily basis and was able to carry out many tasks on a routine basis.

I tried to practise my three "P"s:-

Prioritise Pat's needs when considering future plans or changing circumstances.
Be Proactive in anticipating and pre-empting possible problems
Be Patient in helping Pat cope with PD effects

- and never forget that Pat was the unlucky one, not me.

Pat's Daily Drug Regime			
Medication	**Brand Name**	**Colour**	**Take at:**
Co-Beneldopa 62.5 mg	Madapar	Dispersable	7.00am
Careldopa 25mg/100mg CR	Caramet	Orange	7.30
Amantadine	Symmetrel	Red	7.30
Furosemide (HF)		White	7.30
Mesalazine (UC)	Pentasa	White	9.00
Ropinirole 4mg	Requip	Light Brown	10.00
Levodopa 62.5	Sinemet	Yellow	10.30
Careldopa 25mg/100mg CR	Caramet	Orange	12.30
Amantadine	Symmetrel	Red	12.30
Furosemide 20g (HF)		White	12.30
Levodopa 62.5	Sinemet	Yellow	3.00
Careldopa 25mg/100mg CR	Caramet	Orange	5.00
Amantadine	Symmetrel	Red	5.00

Levodopa 62.5	Sinemet	Yellow	7.00
Mesalazine (UC)	Pentasa	White	9.00
Levodopa 62.5	Sinemet	Yellow	9.00
Candesarta 8mg (HF)	Amias	Pink	Last thing
Ropinirole 8mg	Requip	Light Brown	Last thing

Drugs are for PD except those marked UC for ulcerated colitis and HF for heart failure

~~~~~

Pritam Brar – Carer for Gurdev Brar – PD Client

We came to know about INS in 2007 after a kind social services person told us about INS in Kew. My husband Gurdev Brar had been diagnosed with Parkinson's disease in December 1999.

Since his diagnoses up to 2007 he had been prescribed different medications by different neurologists. In 2007 he had been on pergolide agonists for three years. To begin with this drug was great because physical body functions improve and outwardly the person with Parkinson's looks well, but the adverse psychological effect of this drug is beyond describable.

My husband was not the same person. He was having hallucinations all the time. He was seeing things which I did not understand. He was suspicious of everything all the time. He was changing locks in the house and hiding keys. It was not possible to go for walk with him because he was thinking every person passing us knew me and made eyes at me. I couldn't understand what was happening and what I was supposed to do.

I explained to my GP that I was getting suicidal coping with this behaviour and his reply was this is the effect of the drugs which is normal. but he did not offer me any support or help. His neurologist told me that my husband's brain was playing tricks on him, it was not his fault; it is the effect of the drug agonists. I was hiding in the house for most of the time not knowing what to do.

As soon as the social services told me about INS, I made contact by phone. A kind and helpful voice told me someone from INS would visit
~~~~~

us at our home. We had the visit the same week and were told in detail about the services INS could provide for us.

1. Exercise for my husband to control his Parkinson's deterioration by trained therapists and staff who are so helpful and caring.

He was able to communicate with people in a similar condition. He looked forward to meeting his exercise group every week. This enabled him to get ready in the morning, travelling by car, the whole day became exciting, and gaining valuable experience.

2. Support for me as a carer.

I was listened to with empathy and an understanding of how difficult it was for me to cope with my husband's behaviour under the side effects of the drug agonists. I was offered a 12-week counselling with fully experienced therapist. Counselling healed me and got me out of the dark hole I was stuck in for so long that I even forgot how to smile.

This was only the beginning.

INS opened a whole new way of living and coping with a chronic Parkinson's condition. We carers were offered our own Carer group meeting once a week. In that group we discussed what we faced in our carer role. By sharing our experiences and having discussions we got help and support and found mechanisms for coping in our daily caring duties.

Also, of great help were fitness classes for carers under the supervision of professionals and hydrotherapy sessions for both of us.

A highlight of the year was Christmas Lunch for all members with neurological conditions and their carers. You can understand how uplifting that experience was for both of us. Another great treat was the Boat trip every summer on the river Thames.

It was all provided by INS

INS support was a lifeline for me. The best thing is INS support you all the time at every stage of your condition. After joining INS in 2007 at Kew Baptist church we both received full support from INS till Gurdev's death in September 2017.

After my husband's passing it was INS where I found a way to meet other carers who were in a similar situation. We share our loss and we discuss how we are coping. Something I look forward to is our Mind, Body, and Spirit group which kept going on Zoom during the Covid lockdown.

We discuss every topic, keeping up to date with all members of the group; health well-being, body well-being, spirit well-being. Our members are from every walk of life, like me a former carer, someone with a neurological condition, suffering from Parkinson's, stroke, or MS. We share our well-being and that is such a help to keep going, because there is organisation which is willing to support you, and it is INS.

~~~~~

Anne Foulds – Carer for Mike Foulds – PD Client

Mike was diagnosed with Parkinson's in 1995 after his GP referred him to a consultant at West Middlesex hospital. He was given medication and was also seen at the National Hospital for Neurology and Neurosurgery, Queen Square. There was no support for the family at this time of diagnosis.

The Challenging Journey

Mike and we, his family, had to cope with his increasing lack of mobility and his reluctance to do a regular programme to keep himself fit, especially for his golf, which was a favourite sport. After some years he had increasing falls and he was not very good at doing what he was asked to do! When he needed carers they had no time to encourage him to try to keep himself as strong and mobile as possible to do the things he wanted to do, e.g. move easily or turn over in bed. It was very difficult for him to get in and out of the car.

Later, he was diagnosed with Progressive Supranuclear Palsy (PSP, a rare progressive condition that causes problems with balance, movement, vision, speech, and swallowing) which made him change mood quickly from laughter to tears which was difficult for his family and friends to deal with.

Gradually it became increasingly difficult for him to remain at home after he had a short spell in hospital with a gastric issue and I was recovering from bowel cancer. Of course, we had long family deliberations about this but finally decided it would be for the best for him to move into Lynde House Care Home in 2008, then into Atfield House in 2009 where he died in 2010.
~~~~~

Help from INS

In 1998 Mike was referred to INS through contacts at his Royal Mid-Surrey Golf Club and INS became a great help and support for 12 years of our challenging journey. Ellie came to see us and was incredibly supportive and gave Mike a programme to follow. He joined the INS Parkinson's group which was held weekly, which he really enjoyed along with the occasional outing. Ellie was a frequent visitor, especially when he was diagnosed with PSP and the charity was involved in helping in the needed alterations to the house.

I am still involved with INS as a "Friend of INS", people who help to raise funds and awareness of the charity. I believe INS is a wonderful model of what can be done to alleviate the social and economic burdens of neurological conditions in the UK.

~~~~~
~~~~~

Chapter 4
Volunteers & Social Work

Kate Hodgkinson – Volunteer Befriender

Long before I became personally involved with INS I was well aware of the valued support that close friends with specific problems were receiving from this charitable organisation.

Some years ago INS was located in Kew Baptist Church in Kew, when Dr Liz Grove gave a presentation about the organisation at St Anne's Church in Kew. Dr Grove explained that INS was keen to encourage people to become volunteers in a wide range of activities; e.g. organising outings, fundraising, general support for groups or joining the Befriending team. I felt that I could best help by becoming an official volunteer Befriender.

Dr Grove suggested I might like to become a Befriender for a mutual friend's family as their need for support was increasing. I was very happy to accept. I will always be very grateful for the guidance and encouragement that the INS team gave me. I look back over this period with deep emotion. It was a truly personal and privileged experience to be alongside such a loving Christian family. Our friendship deepened as time went by and now we look back and share many happy memories.

After a brief period, I felt able to be introduced to a new client. June Reid (a fellow Befriender) and I sought approval from INS to visit a new client who had been housebound for years and, with no family, was therefore very isolated. Our client had limited speech, very little mobility and was bed-bound. June and I thought that in these circumstances the extra stimulation would prove beneficial.

It proved so rewarding to see her positive response, huge smile of recognition on our arrival, eye contact that showed understanding and a great sense of humour – we laughed a lot - good therapy for the three of us! Now this lady had been transferred to a Care Home and we continue the same successful regime.

A year ago we became Befrienders to another INS client who had been admitted to the same Care Home. June and I established a happy relationship with our new friend and her family. Sometimes we were able to sit outside in the gardens together for a chat, sharing family joys and sorrows. Now we are looking forward to the arrival of their second grandchild.

We consider we are the fortunate ones, having built up close relationships with our clients and the staff of the Care Home over the years. Our weekly visits are planned ahead and if we are away or unable to visit we contact the Care Home to send our love and make sure all is well.

June and I appreciate the support we receive from the INS team which provides constantly available source of advice.

Regular meetings are held at which we report on our individual clients and benefit from sharing our experiences and concerns with each other. Most important is the friendship INS engenders through its many social events – lectures, Quiz nights, Line Dancing, INS stalls which we help to organise at local fairs held in Twickenham, Kew and Richmond.

Over the years June and I feel privileged to be involved and be part of such an inspirational organisation.

~~~~~

Janet Holmes – Volunteer Befriender

I was introduced to Robbie and Julia by Liz Grove as part of the INS befriending scheme. From then on I used to make weekly visits when I would make tea and chat to them, sometimes easing a tense situation between them.

Robbie was severely disabled as a result of a stroke he suffered some years earlier and used a motorised wheelchair. He had carers twice a day to hoist him in and out of bed. The rest of the time Julia cared for him with great difficulty as she also had suffered a stroke and was partly paralysed down one side. Their living conditions was far from ideal; Robbie had his bed in the sitting room, there was a very small kitchen and between the two there was an area with an open fire which they kept going between them.

There was no downstairs toilet, so every time Robbie wished to empty his bowels he had to take himself into the garage where he was able to stand for a very short time while Julia pulled down his trousers, moved his wheelchair and replaced it with the commode for him to use. When he was ready she had to do it in reverse. I did alter his trousers, so that
~~~~~

instead of having to pull them down she was able to open a flap at the back, but they were not entirely successful.

In December 2004 Julia fell downstairs and was taken to hospital where she was found to have a severe urine infection. This left Robbie on his own and, unfortunately, he could be very difficult and really disliked his social worker so he did not receive all the help he needed or even accept all the help he was offered.

The help he did have was not always satisfactory. I increased my visits and a neighbour sometimes took him meals. I realised how difficult it was for Julia, when on one of my visits he asked me for my help when he wanted to empty his bowels. On one occasion when Robbie was going by taxi to visit Julia in hospital, I arrived before the visit and found him trying to have a shave using cold tea left over from his breakfast. I then gave him a shave as he wanted to look respectable to visit his wife. Fortunately, he welcomed my visits and accepted my help.

It became obvious that Julia would no longer be fit enough to return to the cottage and care for Robbie; their social worker looked for residential care for them and found a double room at a nursing home to be funded by the local council.

Robbie never settled in the nursing home, was very unhappy and, even though the care he was getting was better than he had received for years, his health did not improve. In June 2005 he was taken into St Peter's Hospital where he died. I took Julia to see him some hours before he died. It was obvious to both of us that she would not be seeing him again and that was one of the hardest things I had to do; finding the right time with Julia for her to say goodbye to him.

At Robbie's funeral I met Julia's family and a family member who asked if I would take him and Julia to the solicitors in Teddington where Robbie and Julia had their wills. This we did a couple of weeks later.

Julia needed to make a new will now that Robbie had died. She said she did not know who to leave her money to as she did not think her family needed it. It was suggested that she leave it to charity, so I suggested the two charities that had helped Julia over the years, Homelink and INS. The solicitor and her nephew agreed that it was suitable and Julia was very agreeable. There were also numerous personal items which she wished to bequeath to named members of her family.

In August 2008 Julia had a letter from the local council saying that she owed a large amount of money and threatening court action if she did not pay. I made an appointment to see the council officer responsible and learnt that it had come to light that Robbie and Julia had money in a building society of which the council were not aware. During the meeting I had sight of the assessment form signed by Julia, but obviously, completed by her social worker, who had been given access to all Robbie and Julia's financial details.

The form showed interest from the building society but the capital was not entered. I was told that Julia owed the money as she and Robbie should have been self-funding. I said that if they had been funding themselves their money would have soon been below the threshold and the borough in which they had lived, would have been funding them. I was not prepared for Julia to pay the council the money until I was sure that Julia would be reimbursed by their home borough.

The dispute over funding carried on for months, involving many letters, phone calls and meetings with council officials. Under the Freedom of Information Act I asked to see all the notes made by Robbie and Julia's social worker but the council wrote to say they were not pursuing the debt any further. I kept her nephew informed with all the details of the dispute, sending him copies of the letters.

I continued my frequent visits to Julia at the nursing home, where she was well cared for and, for most of the time, was happy. I did shopping for her when she needed anything. I had regular contact with her nephew and sent him bank statements and details of her expenses.

In 2011 Julia began to show signs of depression and was losing her appetite. After some time she seemed to lose the will to live and refused drinks, the nursing home discussed the situation with me, I felt that she would not wish to be kept alive by force feeding, but it should be discussed with her nephew and the family. All agreed and Julia was allowed to die in October 2011, aged 96. I was with her nearly all of every day for the last few days of her life and she was so loved by all the staff that the Sister and Staff Nurse sat with her during their off duty late evenings.

The last thing I did for Julia was to provide her family with refreshments after her funeral. They all expressed their gratitude for all that had been done for Julia.

Over the seven years I was a befriender to Robbie and latterly just to Julia I could not have done all that without the support and guidance of the INS staff. The befrienders' meetings, where I was able to discuss difficult situations with the staff and other befrienders, were invaluable. The monthly reports were also important to me as I felt that, through the reports, INS knew and, hopefully, approved of all I was doing.

~~~~~

Daphne Jowit – A Volunteer's Impressions

When I started volunteering with the Stroke group at INS I was immediately struck by the unique blend of professionalism, friendliness, and empathy towards the clients. The atmosphere within the group I joined was always cheerful and understanding of the individual and varied needs, and the priority was on attaining a "can do" attitude, with each person being encouraged to develop as normal a pattern of behaviour as was possible.

The day was divided into two, with therapy in the morning using various aids and techniques to stretch and help each person learn how body movements can be more normalised with repetition and conscious awareness. Then after a break for communal lunch the afternoon sessions were a mixture of fun and achievement.

We had music therapy with a wonderful musician who brought in "rain forest" instruments, which were handed out to everyone, so that they could accompany her and use whatever movement and coordination was possible, which obviously varied from person to person. There was also a lovely art teacher, who encouraged all different media, and got Christmas cards made for sale, and paintings produced for an art exhibition. There was even a term of mosaic making, resulting in a beautiful wall plaque to hang in the building.

We also had many baking afternoons, ranging from Christmas cakes to fruit salads, buns and biscuits, and pizzas, so that the clients could take the results of their labours home to enjoy with their families.

These activities were so much more rewarding than simply doing exercises for the sake of them. We had gardening and sewing groups, too, and one particularly enjoyable activity was when the clients were invited to bring memorabilia to the group and we were able to piece together a life story for each of them, using memory triggers to help them.
~~~~~

Sometimes we went on outings: to Richmond Park, the river, and to exhibitions, and we had picnics and the occasional parties, with lots of fun and laughter.

Over the years the group became closer, with each member having something unique to bring to the friendships, and no one feeling left out - and there was always an open welcome for newcomers.

INS offered so much more than the professional help of therapy, important as it was - members were seen very much as normal people with a particular set of problems that needed some help to minimise or overcome.

I'm sure the members looked forward to their Thursday meetings with as much enthusiasm as I did! I was very disappointed when they changed their day to a Tuesday, as I was no longer able to be part of the group. I had come to care very much about each and every one of them, and being a volunteer was a life-changing experience for me, as I learned so much about how easy - and wrong - it is to judge people by appearances.

The volunteers were given some interesting experiences, like being wheeled down the street in a wheelchair to make us realise how vulnerable it feels, and we were trained to help the clients to do as much for themselves as possible, without interfering but always being on hand. I remember some occasions when I had to stand and watch as one tried to struggle into a coat, and I wanted so much to help, but knew it was important to give them the chance to do it for themselves, even if it took a long time. It was so rewarding to see the sense of achievement when they realised they could actually do something that they thought was no longer possible.

~~~~~

Caroline Hill – Reflections on my Experiences at INS as a Trustee and then as a Volunteer

As far as I know, INS is one of a kind. I am not aware of any other charity that offers what it does – a 'wrap-around' package that aims to support the whole person in whatever ways they need, as they face the challenge of life-changing illnesses such as Parkinson's disease, multiple sclerosis (MS), stroke or other long-term degenerative neurological conditions.

The impact is huge, and because of the degenerative nature of many of the conditions, likely to become more marked over time, threatening
~~~~~

every aspect of daily life - getting up out of bed, washing, dressing; eating drinking preparing food; walking, balance, getting out and about to do the things they have always done and enjoyed, meeting friends, going to work. Financial insecurity. Increasing dependence on the help of others to live their 'normal' life, diminishing quality of life, the uncertainties of the 'road map' of their future life's pathway following what to many will be a devastating diagnosis. Anxiety, fear, and loss – loss of the person they once were, the life they once led.

After the first shock ... what next? What will happen? Who to turn to for help? What help is available? And if this is what INS clients are thinking .... what about their families, spouses, friends, carers? You do not get training to prepare for this.

INS's response is to step in to answer some of these questions, and to provide profession-led treatment, information and advice, practical assistance, emotional support and opportunities to meet other people – to clients, and importantly to family and carers. INS provides interventions that help at a symptomatic level – movement, balance, avoiding falls, poor sleep, communication difficulties; practical interventions and adaptations in the home, help applying for benefits, emotional and psychological support, information and education, and as important, meeting others – making new friends among people who understand what has happened to them, but also being able to help by sharing experiences. A whole range of leisure activities – gardening, arts and crafts, music, creative writing. Showing clients that you do not have to give up on all your interests and the things you liked doing just because of this... but just maybe, you need help learning how to adapt them so that you can still enjoy doing them.

But as well as helping its clients with symptomatic relief, I think INS is doing something else. Its aim is to help people maintain their independence and optimal quality of life for as long as is practicable given the nature of their condition. I would suggest that in providing this holistic, integrated 'wrap around' service, helping the individual as a whole, it is giving its clients much needed confidence to manage their condition.

Psychological research literature would suggest that confidence in managing stressful events – and the diagnosis of a degenerative neurological condition is certainly going to be one of these - is associated with a more positive outcome – and for INS clients, this means maintaining their independence and quality of life as long as is practicable given their condition.

People who cope better with stress are those who feel they have what they need – that is, they have the "resources" they need to help them manage. These can be anything - having the physical ability, the emotional stability, the financial security, the knowledge, the skills required, the social support networks in place. "Resources" are whatever it is a person needs to help them manage in a time of crisis. Having the resources enables them to grow in confidence that they can cope. This in turn helps them manage better, and they have better outcomes. These are often seen in terms of better quality of life.

While I was a volunteer at INS, I had an opportunity to explore some of these ideas as part of a Master's degree at St George's Medical School. My study with clients with Parkinson's disease was limited and only a first step. But its findings supported the suggestion that those who felt more confident they could cope, and who were active in managing their condition, would have better outcomes in terms of quality of life.

This was very gratifying because it fitted in with my experience of clients at INS – and of their carers. Not only were clients getting symptomatic relief, they were being helped to gain confidence that they could manage the challenges they were facing.

It would be good to see more charities like INS offering similar services to other people who would benefit from this kind of help and care.

~~~~~

Carol Williams – Social Worker

Client A had a stroke which gave her left side paralysis and dysarthria (difficulty in speaking clearly due to muscle weakness). She was able to go home six months later to a second floor flat with no lift, where she lived with her fiancé. She was referred to INS.

She had been a bus driver until her stroke and had to give up her job. Her fiancé, also a bus driver, gave up his job to become her carer.

She was finding it difficult to cope emotionally and physically. She had had some bad experiences whilst in hospital and following her discharge from other organisations. When the initial assessment was carried out by myself a month after her return home she was feeling worthless and very worried about the future. It was difficult for them to leave the flat due to
~~~~~

the two flights of stairs; her mobility was poor and she needed to mobilise in her wheelchair.

Her fiancé, now her carer, mentioned to me that they were looking to move, but there was nothing available that was suitable for their needs via the local authority. Their current landlord was unhelpful. They were feeling very demoralised with the lack of help and support they were getting.

In my position as a social worker with INS, I had regular contact with local charities who support local residents and I had just received information about a new build in the local area; a charity was looking for suitable people with a disability to move into a two bedroomed, ground floor flat. I was able to give client and carer the information. They decided to apply and were invited to move in a few weeks later.

This transformed their lives. They have been able to do so much together that was a struggle before. When client A had her stroke, they had been about to get married. They had cancelled the wedding. After moving into their new home and feeling so much better in all respects, they did get married. Her self-esteem and confidence increased dramatically; her partner felt much better supported and happy to know they could come to INS for support and help when needed. Client A has now started to join other groups in the area.

Both benefited from the services and support that INS offer. As social worker, I was able to coordinate the other services that were available and suitable for both, signposting and ensuring that colleagues at INS could offer appropriate groups/support as available and needed. They also benefited from meeting other clients and carers. Her husband/ carer joined a carer group that I coordinated; a group that several years later still meets regularly to support each other.

I consider that I have been so lucky to work for INS to support clients and carers in ways that I would not have been able to do with a statutory service. My time is not limited with clients. I can be available for them whenever a crisis or other issue occurs without having to go through what can often be a difficult referral process. I can work with them freely to give them the tools to be independent and maintain their independence.

There are few bureaucracy or budgetary implications. I can do social work which I have been trained to do. I can work within a multi-disciplinary team which works very well together and upholds the ethos of INS to work holistically with clients and carers.

~~~~~
~~~~~

Chapter 5
Living with Parkinson's – The Road Ahead

David Beales

LIVING WITH PARKINSON'S

Since my formal diagnosis of Parkinson's (PD) in August 2017 preceded by seven years of very early signs, I retired and find myself on the other side of the desk from my previous work, as a General Practitioner. I had also been a physician and specialist with a particular interest in elderly care. [1] Little did I know the challenges of living with a longstanding neurological illness. Now at 78 years of age, I hope this personal account will encourage other people, living with PD, either as patient or supporter, to continue to live well and not be dominated by PD.

My Experience at Time of Diagnosis

The diagnosis was finally made by a consultant neurologist in Southampton in August 2017, privately, having been wrongly treated by a consultant rheumatologist with steroids for a condition called polymyalgia rheumatica, and facing a five-month waiting list to see an NHS neurologist. At the time I thought the process seemed very mechanistic. My history revealed increasing muscle stiffness for three years which had been preceded by unexplained symptoms of sleep disturbance with vivid dreams where I acted as if the dream was affecting me directly. On one occasion I threw myself out of bed when dreaming I was being pursued by assassins. These symptoms are called: type 2 sleep disorder (seven years); shoulder stiffness (five years); severe constipation (one and a half years); slower walking (two years); and excessive sleepiness by day (two years).

Testing revealed stiff muscles of a particular type called cogwheeling, and walking speed was diminished with reduced arm swing. Parkinson's named. I was given a prescription for L-Dopa (Levodopa) tablets followed by goodbye and see you for follow-up in three months. Support services were only briefly mentioned. I left the appointment in shock, later bursting into tears in the car park.

Ripples

A poem written by me following my diagnosis with Parkinson's.

In time age gathers momentum
Muscles feel stiff and energy dips
Love of life keeps my spirits up
Counting my blessings guides me still.

Each new day has an ebb and flow
I wait for the rip tide to pull me under
Just breathe and with each breath
Return to firm ground once more.

Staying alive to love and live
Ripples of calm to rise and fall
New birth to celebrate afresh
And my stiffness has a name.

Parkinson's makes sense of small steps
Stiff shoulders and energy dips
Not a name that conjures magic
But finally, to understand and tame.

Discoveries and Learning: Four and a Half Years Since Formal Diagnosis

James Parkinson described the "shaking palsy" in 1817, and since then both clinicians and patients have hoped for a curative medication; none exists so far. As research progressed findings showed that cells within the brain producing the chemical messenger Dopamine had died, accumulating in some people with Parkinson's an abnormal protein called alpha synuclein which stops the cell functioning. Dopamine helps coordinate movement in different parts of the body. A much more detailed account of the detailed brain pathways involved can be found at the Science of Parkinson's website. [2]

Disease modifying agents have emerged as well as drugs to stimulate the production of Dopamine, particularly L-Dopa which was discovered in 1910. The first study reporting improvements in patients with Parkinson's disease resulting from treatment with L-Dopa was published in 1968. Dopamine deficiency throughout the body-mind system (particularly in the centre's controlling movement called the substantia nigra) is thought to be the root cause of many symptoms particularly slowness of movement.

I was initially prescribed L-Dopa as Sinemet Plus 100/25mg four times daily which I discontinued for two and a half years before restarting two years ago. During this time, I changed my food habits and added Curcumin – a desert spoonful daily with breakfast – [3] and took care to introduce a vegetable dominant diet with extra fibre as Normacol one sachet twice daily, regular vigorous exercise, and stretch programmes which I will go on to describe. Two years ago, I went back to L-Dopa – as Sinemet Plus 100/25mg four times daily a half hour before food. Additional medications include Rotigotine 1mg daily, Selegiline 1mg daily

One of my main concerns has been the importance of understanding the actions, typical doses, and side effects of PD medication.

Since L-Dopa was initially so effective at restoring Dopamine levels, it has become the drug often offered as first choice on diagnosis. However, with accumulated doses, side effects (caused by the production of 3-O-Methyldopa created by prolonged use), are thought to reduce the effectiveness and tolerance. L-Dopa is usually combined with a Decarboxylase inhibitor. This group of medications reduces adverse effects enabling L-Dopa to cross the barrier between the brain and body.

Despite this, 90% of oral L-Dopa is metabolised to 3-O-Methyldopa. Escalating requirements and on/off fluctuations are then often ascribed to these progressive increases in dose rather than the possibility of side effects. Unwanted body and facial muscle movements outside the control of the conscious mind occur, called Dyskinesia. These abnormal movements, often accompanied by sudden freezing of body movement, may be interpreted as due to progression rather than medication. [4]

I discovered these facts gradually and stopped L-Dopa substituting drugs to increase the availability of Dopamine being produced in adequate quantities within my body-mind system. I returned to taking L-Dopa two years further on, after these drugs became less effective. I now take L-Dopa 100mg four times a day with Amantadine 100mg twice daily and Rotigotine (Neupro) 8mg as a patch once daily.

Dr John Dobbs and colleagues discuss these issues in their paper, The Case of Tolerance to L-Dopa. [5] The authors make the case to resist the early use of L-Dopa because of issues of tolerance and the toxicity due to

3-O-Methyldopa. Others [6] demonstrate that 3-O-Methyldopa accumulation from long-term L-Dopa treatment may be involved in the adverse effects of L-Dopa therapy.

I needed to be bold when first offered this drug and bring up issues relating to tolerance, side effects and dependency relating to L-Dopa use. This should have been discussed before the almost automatic prescription when first diagnosed.

When I realised these implications, after seeing John and Sylvia Dobbs at King's College as part of their research, I stopped L-Dopa and followed their recommendations for other medication such as Neupro (Rotigotine). I later added UDCA (Uro-Deoxy-Cholic Acid) 1g twice daily whilst awaiting the results of a randomised controlled trial of UDCA versus placebo.

I restarted L-Dopa building up to my present dose of 100mg four times daily, a half hour before food, two years ago. I have not noticed Dyskinesia or on/off symptoms. My body control remains good, and I can briskly walk for 5km as well as play tennis.

In summary: I learned that increasing intake of L-Dopa may lead to abnormal movements (on/off movements/Dyskinesia) resulting from side effects of medication. As tolerance to L-Dopa increases so the likelihood of these difficult-to-manage side-effects increases, and need be distinguished from progression of the disease itself. [7]

I think that the holistic approaches I adopted – exercise, nutrition to build a healthy microbiome, enjoyment of an active life with hobbies and tennis has helped me to live purposely and with enjoyment. I live with Parkinson's and am not dominated by the condition.

This makes it even more important to look for evidence-based approaches involving the whole mind-body network, such as exercise and nutrition at the beginning of the journey involved in living with Parkinson's. Daily exercise including high intensity programmes with conscious regular walking has been shown to slow progression by up to 40%. John Pepper details his recovery from diagnostically proven PD in the book *The Brain's Way of Healing* by Norman Doidge (Chapter 2, How conscious walking helps fend off degenerative disorders). In this chapter, he describes how he "walked off" his Parkinson's symptoms. [8]

One of my main concerns has been the importance of fully understanding the actions and side effects of PD medication.

The Need for an Integrated Approach

Parkinson's affects many different systems of the body and for any individual there is no single discipline that combats the disease. The disciplines needed may include, for example, vascular medicine, gastroenterology, pulmonology, neuro-ophthalmology, urology, geriatric/elderly care, palliative care, and dentistry.

It thus makes sense to introduce a community based multi-disciplinary model for living with Parkinson's. Such an integrated approach is promoted by the consultant neurologist Bastiaan Bloem [9] in Holland and supported by Steve Ford (previously chief executive of Parkinson's UK) and put into practice at the European Parkinson Therapy Centre in Italy. [10]

The Importance of Exercise

Modern research has found evidence that the brain is able to re-wire itself following damage. This is called neuroplasticity, also known as neural plasticity, or brain plasticity, and is the ability of neural networks in the brain to change through growth and reorganisation.

The brain continues to create new neuro pathways and alter existing ones to adapt to new experiences, learn new information and create new memories. Lockwood, Klein and Robbins have provided evidence that exercise enhances the limbic system functioning which has been damaged in Parkinson's. [11]

Movement is coordinated by the limbic system which integrates various centres within the brain, communicating closely with the basal ganglia. These centres support and control voluntary movement, cognitive planning, emotions, and rewards, as well as cognition and learning [12]

Enhancing neuroplasticity is an essential part of stabilizing your condition. Very important work by Becky Farley [13] on neuroplasticity demonstrates the value of enhancing new pathways within the brain and body, to bring back functions that have been temporarily lost in PD.

Brief intermittent high-intensity exercise (HIT) which raises the pulse rate to two thirds of its maximum, leads to the increased release of brain stimulating hormone and enhances the impact of exercise on your plasticity. I recently bought an exercise bicycle which I use daily following an exercise protocol.

The aim for me and perhaps you, is to be one's own coach. This includes following through on changing lifestyle and habits, as well as keeping enough energy in reserve. I (alongside colleagues) have described a method in our book, *Reclaim Health,* [14] using self-monitoring by our observing self to stick to exercise routines.

Many of us need enhanced support with an encourager or trainer. Ellie Kinnear (the co-founder of INS) and myself believe that enhanced support to carry out a structured movement programme is very effectively provided by a conductive educator. The conductive approach to neuroplasticity has been demonstrated to enhance movement and muscle control and is provided at NICE (National Institute of Conductive Education) in Birmingham. I undertook an online Zoom class which was helpful. [15]

Exercise in Practice

• I believe one of the essential needs in PD is for a tailor-made exercise programme with a daily routine. This would include high intensity exercise alongside stretch and resistance elements, as well as dexterity and balance.

• Brisk walking under conscious control has been shown to reverse PD. Be careful pacing activities and ensure you have adequate rest between sessions. Conscious walking where I use my gluteal muscles (situated around our backside and engaged in standing from a sitting position to launch the step) needs to be strengthened. The value of Nordic walking to get the feel of this change in walking action is helpful. I try and fit in an hour of brisk walking three times a week.

• Listen to the body and mind. For me, this involves slowing down and thinking out an achievable focus for each day.

• I still find it difficult to channel my frustration and find a balance between acceptance of the disease and actively resisting giving in to muscle stiffness and disability.

• High-intensity training at high energy using an exercise bicycle is of great value. A 2016 study found that a ten-minute workout with just one minute of high intensity (in this case, sprinting), had the same benefits as 45 minutes of jogging.

I use an exercise bicycle. I find that two minutes intensive exercise raising my heart rate to 80% of maximum, followed by gentle idling for two minutes and then repeating intermittently for 20 minutes suits me well.

- When walking, I need to be aware if I am using my back to lever my movement/momentum, rather than my gluteal muscles. The aim is to achieve lift off whilst initiating a walking step. Vigilance and conscious application of these principles will take concentration. An OptoGait analysis helped. [16]

Balance measurements confirmed that I was favouring my right side (the left is more rigid with cogwheeling).

I haven't been helped to deconstruct my walking style. This is something that would be useful, in order to replace it with one that is conscious and reproducible.

Communication

Speech: I need to practise regular speech exercises to avoid my tendency to slur my speech. This would involve slowing down, being mindful of what I want to say, then breaking the speech into chunks. Speech therapy is essential and I also need to practise my voice exercises every morning.

Handwriting: I have been given handwriting exercises to help me address my present problem of handwriting becoming smaller and more illegible.

Psychological

My chief aim is to live with PD rather than being dominated by PD. Not be defined by the disease. Be kind to myself. Live with gratitude with compassion to self and others.

In summary, what I need to bring into my life living side-by-side with Parkinson's and so that it doesn't take over my life are: awareness, acceptance, and action/practice.

Awareness: our automatic patterns of feeling, thinking, and behaving when faced with a serious disease like Parkinson's may cause us to fall asleep to our own lives. In ongoing research, 60% of us will become depressed and anxious during its course. Rather than staying in automatic mode, PD is a call to wake up by learning how to observe and study myself/ourselves more objectively. Staying well with PD means that I/we need to become more aware of our automatic reactions. Then we see that

I/we have no option other than to behave and react differently with compassion for ourselves.

Acceptance: adopt a kinder and more caring attitude toward myself and others and accept what arises in the moment. I know I need to accept my reactivity and a tendency to drive myself. Accept my frustration in owning and defending this part of myself which has proved useful in the past but can now drive me to do too much too long which worsens my PD symptoms.

Action/Practice: noticing my body-mind reactivity, I have observed that the first thing that happens when I become frustrated is that my body tightens and I become defensive. Is it any wonder that stress/overload makes the Parkinson's worse! I know that paying attention to my breath pattern and staying with the out-breath whilst slowing it down takes me to a calm space of peace within. Using a Neurosteer device [17], which showed the alpha waves as I moved into this calm state was helpful. There are also many aids to creating calm such as meditation using exercises. These can be found online, provided by many different companies.

Mindfulness revisited: I know I need to practise awareness and self-acceptance. I need to pay attention to everyday tasks such as cooking a meal, cleaning my teeth, doing up buttons etc. These are mindful tasks to carry out with full attention. There are many times when I feel annoyed at my slowness and stiffness.

Focussing on the breath brings me to accept the present moment – without judgement. Practise conscious awareness of the moment by focusing on your breath and on the primary sensations you are experiencing, without any judgement of those sensations.

The above points show a logical reason for why mindfulness meditation could help reduce not only stress, but also symptoms of Parkinson's by reducing additional inner tension. Becoming present in what I am doing in the moment, assisted by awareness helps in walking consciously. Notice with compassion the body-mind reaction, pause, notice the energy in my body, be present for it. If I notice tightness, loosen its grip by conscious breathing, pause and let go, leading to conscious actions.

Lifestyle

Nutritional: In my journey, PD started in the gut. An initial dietary review by nutritional consultant Karina Athwal was extremely helpful. This led to the treatment of a gut infection with Helicobacter Pylori which stabilised the PD after I received the results of a full microbiota investigation. This further led me to seek out Sylvia and John Dodds (Consultants in Applied Pharmacology) who were running a research trial looking at gut microbes in people with PD and their wives or partners as controls at King's College Hospital in London.

Enjoyment: Being able to retain enjoyment of tennis, yoga, vigorous walking, and a variety of hobbies, such as watercolour painting, has become a priority. Courses in mindfulness and cognitive behavioural therapy (CBT) followed as well as joining the Mind, Body, and Spirit group at INS.

Finding Services and Support

The time to review chronic illness is limited within our NHS. Despite this, since moving from Hampshire to Kew Gardens, I have found services to reduce the impact of Parkinson's in my life. I am not told about them by health professionals, instead seeking them out through enquiry in the locality.

In Hampshire and at INS, I found the PD Warrior exercise classes. This consisted of ten sessions and introduced me to a routine of stretching and vigorous exercise. [18]

There was an excellent Parkinson's nurse at Winchester Hospital and Kew. The research programme running at King's Hospital managed by Sylvia and John Dobbs, looking at the microbiome in people with Parkinson's and their partners was helpful. I had already confirmed that I was carrying Helicobacter Pylori in my gut which was treated and eradicated. This is an added risk factor for Parkinson's. The Parkinson's UK website and patient forums were invaluable.

After moving to Kew in London two and a half years ago and contacting Nick Ephgrave from Parkinson's UK, I found INS exercise and physiotherapy sessions, a variety of courses, the friendship and support of INS co-founder Ellie Kinnear, a local gym (The Cambrian – with a trainer), a PD nurse, nutritional advice from Karina Athwal and the great support of the Avenue Club men's group in Kew led by Gary Freer.

I am so grateful for the loving support of family, my life partner Helen Whitten, friends particularly Gary and all in the Avenue Club Kew men's group, Phil, Charlie, Ellie and the Mind, Body, and Spirit group at INS and many other supporters, including the European Parkinson's Therapy Centre. I attended for a week in September 2021 in Italy which was invaluable. [19]

My Involvement with Support

When I moved from Hampshire two and a half years ago, I recognised the need for an integrated programme to preserve function in PD. Having been told about INS by Parkinson's UK I self-referred. I took part in an exercise class called PD Warrior once weekly for eight weeks and joined the Mind, Body, and Spirit group and taking part in group discussions every two weeks.

I first went to INS for the exercise class as a stand-alone. However, as my needs became more apparent, I was helped to adjust my exercise routine after a physiotherapy assessment and the Mindfulness course.

I have also been impressed by a weekly programme run by 4D Life encompassing many of the features described above, and by a more comprehensive exercise regime to improve movement of the fingers particularly, run by the National Institute of Conductive Education. After giving up voice recognition, in frustration, I have returned to touch typing.

Subsequently, I have had an excellent Zoom consultation with Mary-Anne (the physiotherapist at INS) which resulted in me altering my exercise routine. It will help me to have a key worker and a yearly needs assessment.

Condition Today

Today I am independent, walk 5,000 steps with ease, enjoy life including tennis, holidays abroad and at home, painting, and writing. I further cherish a loving relationship with my partner Helen, a family of four sons and their partners/wives with eight grandchildren.

This is not to say that I do not feel terribly frustrated at times by slowness of movement and problems with doing up buttons and shoelaces. I feel most alive when playing tennis when my body just gets into gear, and I can hit the ball without knowing quite how I got there.

Muscle memory kicks in automatically and I now know that walking needs to be conscious rather than automatic.

This medicine cocktail is combined with a high fibre diet rich in vegetables and fruits aiming for 30g a day of fibre. I've been able to reduce or eliminate laxatives. I know not to take L-Dopa within half an hour of eating food and have an alarm prompt on my iPhone so the four times a day dosage is reliably met.

I get going with an exercise routine for each morning including stretches and weights, walk each day including a long walk three times week. I love painting watercolours with an excellent teacher. [20]

THE ROAD AHEAD: HOW MATTERS CAN BE IMPROVED

Better Information at Time of Diagnosis

This would include aspects such as:

- More explanation and information about likely causation and pathology. After a brief consultation I was given L-Dopa as Sinemet-Plus 100/25 four times daily without any further information.

- To know that the course of the disease is very individual, with up to 50 subtypes.

- My estimated length of life is not altered by the diagnosis but the quality will be affected unless I take care and have an active programme to re-establish new pathways through neuroplasticity.

- That treatment needs to be tailor-made to the individual.

- That there are evidence-based strategies and services available to support staying well with Parkinson's rather than the fear of inevitable decline.

- For my partner Helen to have been more involved in the explanation with information on support for her.

- Not to wait six months for diagnosis on the NHS.

The NICE (National Institute from Health and Care Excellence) guidelines are not clear about the need for early assessment following referral by the GP. The recommendation is "soon", which is interpreted by the Provider trust as within six months. After my diagnosis, I wrote to the lead neurologist at Basingstoke Hospital, only to be told that there was no reason for early referral because PD was "incurable, degenerative and progressive".

The Chief Executive of the NHS Trust confirmed this view in a letter to my MP after I complained about the long wait for a consultation on the NHS resulting in a private consultation. This policy is wrong because PD effects can be mitigated, countered, and delayed, if action is taken early.

What Needs to Change?

- At diagnosis, a full assessment should be undertaken. This is described in the First Steps course which has been researched and confirmed as valuable by Parkinson's UK and Oxford Brookes University.

- Early intervention and support in the early stages of diagnosis could save governments millions of pounds.

- I think that early needs assessment must be offered, including a full multi-disciplinary review covering muscle movement, walking, exercise, nutrition, stress management, leading to a personalised activity/action plan.

- To have a personal health record that moves with me and details who is involved in my treatment plan for me to self-monitor my journey.

The Importance of First Steps Following Diagnosis

The First Steps course is currently under study by leading researchers. Initial results show exciting and novel evidence for the impact of a peer led psycho-educational intervention for people newly diagnosed with PD. It supports the notion that positive stories from peers can support and encourage positive attitudes towards behavioural change. [21]

Without early intervention, the newly diagnosed client may lose hope. In a group discussion after a PD Warrior session, I was told, by a newly diagnosed woman, that she went home after the diagnosis to find that her husband had packed his bags and left, leaving her with two small children and enormous stress.

The First Steps course is offered in the UK by Parkinson's UK. The course programme is designed to help people take the first steps in processing their diagnosis and finding out about the information and support available to them to help them live well with Parkinson's. It has been developed with people affected by Parkinson's and is delivered by volunteer hosts who live with the condition.

The programme provides people with the opportunity to meet other people who have a new diagnosis of Parkinson's. Within the groups, people can ask questions, share experiences, take part in group discussions, and hear from other people in a similar situation. Some people attend First Steps with a member of their family or a friend, other people attend on their own.

Guidelines Must be Improved and Implemented

The present NHS guidelines from NICE suggest that people with Parkinson's should receive specialist review at least every six months, usually provided by a consultant and community Parkinson's disease nurse specialist (PDNS).

Despite these recommendations, a recent audit of patient experience found that 46% have consultant appointments delayed by more than six months, and 60% have not seen the community nurse within the last year. Some regions of the UK don't have a specialist service, and 50% of vacant PDNS posts are due to long-term sick leave or resignation. [22]

Treatment Needs to be Personalised

We are still looking for:

1. A disease halting mechanism
2. A neuroprotective agent
3. Some form of restorative therapy

As discussed in a recent article from the Science of Parkinson's Trust: [23]

A curative therapy for Parkinson's is going to need to be personalised to each individual, with varying levels of each of the three-component listed above. It will be a multi-modal approach, designed to best fit each person's needs.

There is a great deal of heterogeneity (or variability) between individuals with regards to their Parkinson's symptoms and the amount of time that they have had the condition. No two cases of Parkinson's are the same. Some people are more tremor dominant, while others do not experience tremor at all. Likewise, some individuals have only just been diagnosed, while others have lived with the condition for many years.

As a result, the treatment needs of each individual will be different, and thus what we will require is differing amounts of each component for each individual. By this I mean, that someone who has only just been diagnosed may only need the disease halting mechanism component, while someone who has had the condition for many years will need different amounts of all three components (depending on their situation).

Treatment Must be Integrated

Integrated treatment and support programmes in the treatment of Parkinson's will be encouraged by the new NHS reforms discussed in the White Paper. [24] For efficiency and cost reasons there is need to pool expertise. A multi-disciplinary team is needed.

Consider the following observations, made in the article Recommendations for the Organization of Multi-disciplinary Clinical Care Teams in the Journal of Parkinson's Disease. [25]

PD is a complex, multi-dimensional condition with cognitive, psychological and social ramifications, as well as motor and non-motor signs. The clinical manifestations are only partially amenable to pharmacological or surgical treatment. This makes it impossible for one healthcare professional in any discipline to cover all. complexities and diversities of symptoms and to deliver all options.

The most important recommendations are: care is organised in a patient-centred way; every newly diagnosed patient has access to a core multi-disciplinary team; and each team has a coordinator.

The following healthcare professionals are part of the core care team: the dietician, movement disorder neurologist, occupational therapist, Parkinson's disease nurse specialist (this may also be a nurse practitioner or registered nurse), physiotherapist, psychiatrist or (neuro)psychologist, social worker and the speech and language therapist. Other healthcare professionals are available for referral

It is essential that one of the patient's care team is the team coordinator. Care coordination is of critical importance in all disease stages as a patient's needs change.

A key issue is bringing the different agencies and disciplines together quickly enough to create an individualised care plan. To do this, it is necessary to ensure that each patient has one key worker assigned to them as well as a comprehensive health record book.

In a similar way, the Department of Health currently insists that over 75s have a single GP accountable for their care. There is much evidence that in complex disease management continuity of care is essential.

Concluding Remarks

When I was the other side of the desk as a practising GP, I set up an audit in practice of those with disability including the over 75-year-olds. Studies were published including one entitled Meeting the needs of disabled people in general practice from 16 to 74 years old. [26] The study found that unmet need was largely linked with social requirements. 49% of all respondents identified areas of unmet need. 28% of carers said they were having difficulties. 18% said their housing had steps causing problems. 82.5% were unhappy with the employment situation. 20% said they wanted someone to talk about their problems. 27% said they were lonely.

I suspect that findings today in most general practices would find similar results. Although social prescribing (lifestyle programmes such as "walking in nature") is a step in the right direction to bridge the gap between medical condition and social support.

The first point of contact is usually the general practitioner, who will receive confirmation of the diagnosis after referral to a consultant neurologist, with a special interest in movement disorders. This is a time to step back with the patient with PD and their supports and create an action plan following a needs assessment.

Integrated centres like INS can do this well and offer ongoing long-term assessment and support following the diagnosis of Parkinson's and other long-term neurological conditions.

REFERENCES

[1] *Community Care for Older People*, Radcliffe. Full biography at: https://drdavidbeales.com

[2] *Dopamine*, The Science of Parkinson's https://scienceofparkinsons.com/dopamine/

[3] Eslam El Nebrisi, *Neuroprotective Activities of Curcumin in Parkinson's Disease*, International Journal of Molecular Sciences, 2021, 22, 11248 https://www.ncbi.nlm.nih.gov/pmc/articles/PMC8537234/

[4] *L-DOPA*, ScienceDirect https://www.sciencedirect.com/topics/neuroscience/l-dopa

[5] R. J. Dobbs et al, *Time-Lag between Establishing Clinical Pharmacology Principles and Advances in Practice: The Case of Tolerance to L-Dopa,* Journal of Pharmacology & Clinical Toxicology, 2017, 5(5): 1084, 2017 https://www.jscimedcentral.com/Pharmacology/pharmacology-5-1084.pdf

Dyskinesia, ScienceDirect, Elsevier https://www.sciencedirect.com/topics/neuroscience/dyskinesia

[6] Eun-Sook Y. Lee, Hongtao Chen, Jennifer King, Clivel Charlton, *The Role of 3-O-Methyldopa in the Side Effects of L-Dopa,* Neurochemical Research, 2008, Vol. 33, pp401–411 https://pubmed.ncbi.nlm.nih.gov/17713853/

[7] *3-O-Methyldopa (3-OMD),* Wikipedia https://en.wikipedia.org/wiki/3-O-Methyldopa

[8] Norman Doidge, *The Brain's Way of Healing,* Allen Lane, 2015

[9] *Professor Bastiaan Bloem & Ending Parkinson's,* Davis Phinney Foundation, October 2020 https://davisphinneyfoundation.org/professor-bastiaan-bloem-ending-parkinsons/

[10] The European Parkinson Therapy Centre https://www.terapiaparkinson.it/en/

[11] *Principles of Experience-Dependent Neural Plasticity: Implications for Rehabilitation After Brain Damage,* Journal of Speech, Language, and Hearing Research, Vol. 51, S225–S239, February 2008 https://www.jsmf.org/meetings/2008/may/Kleim%20&%20Jones%202008.pdf

[12] James Sonne, Vamsi Reddy, Morris R. Beato, *Neuroanatomy, Substantia Nigra,* StatPearls, 2021 https://www.ncbi.nlm.nih.gov/books/NBK536995/

[13] Google Scholar, Becky Farley, NeuroFit Networks DBA Parkinson Wellness Recovery https://scholar.google.com/citations?user=niJTMaEAAAAJ&hl=en

[14] *Reclaim Health*, 2019, available on Amazon. Reclaim Health enables us to step back and engage our "observing self" to co-create our living with PD plan and where exercise fits into it with practical action.

[15] NICE – Centre for Movement Disorders https://conductive-education.org.uk/

[16] OptoGait http://www.optogait.com/

[17] *Neurosteer: Introducing a Novel Brain Activity Monitor*, Health Europa https://www.healtheuropa.eu/brain-activity-neurosteer/88769/

[18] *PD Warrior* is an exercise philosophy designed to help you slow your Parkinson's down https://pdwarrior.com/

[19] The European Parkinson Therapy Centre https://www.terapiaparkinson.it/en/

[20] Frank Walters. Zoom Watercolour Lessons – Workshops, Courses, Holidays https://www.frankwatercolours.com/

[21] *A Qualitative Study on the Impact of First Steps – A Peer-led Educational Intervention for People Newly Diagnosed with Parkinson's Disease*, Behavioral Sciences, 2019, 9, 107 https://www.ncbi.nlm.nih.gov/pmc/articles/PMC6826464/

A qualitative study on the impact of First Steps – a peer-led, educational intervention for people newly diagnosed with Parkinson's Disease, University of Plymouth, 2019 https://pearl.plymouth.ac.uk/bitstream/handle/10026.1/14958/First%20Ste0Accepted%20Version.pdf?sequence=1&isAllowed=y

The course is offered in the UK by Parkinson's UK https://www.parkinsons.org.uk/professionals/first-steps-people-newly-diagnosed-parkinsons

[22] UK Parkinson's Audit – Transforming Care https://www.parkinsons.org.uk/professionals/uk-parkinsons-audit-transforming-care

[23] From *The Road Ahead* a detailed review by the scientific lead for The Science of Parkinson's Trust https://scienceofparkinsons.com/2021/01/25/road-2021/

[24] Helen McKenna, *The health and social care White Paper explained*, The King's Fund, March 2021
https://www.kingsfund.org.uk/publications/health-social-care-white-paper-explained

[25] *Recommendations for the Organization of Multidisciplinary Clinical Care Teams in Parkinson's Disease*, Journal of Parkinson's Disease, July 2020, 10(3): 1087–1098
https://www.ncbi.nlm.nih.gov/pmc/articles/PMC7415700/

[26] G. Parker, D. L. Beales, *Meeting the needs of disabled people in general practice from 16-74 years old,* Professional Nurse, September 1993

~~~~~
~~~~~

PART 3

GOOD PRACTICE & ADVANCES

Chapter 6
Neuroplasticity – Restoring Function in Stroke, Parkinson's, & Other Neurological Conditions

Understanding Neuroplasticity

Neuroplasticity is the name used to describe the capacity of the brain to build new cells (neurons) and the pathways that connect them. New brain cells are encouraged to grow and bypass damaged areas, caused by injury and neurological conditions.

The brain transmits and stores thoughts, emotions, speech, and behaviour together with messages for physical actions and movements by using these neural pathways and storage cells. Effective reablement strategies are designed to encourage neuroplasticity. These are best started as close as possible to the onset of the neurological event.

- The brain can make new connections between brain cells after an injury such as a stroke

- These can be stimulated, for example, by repetitive movements of an affected limb. [See below]

Conditions that reduce movement and balance as in Parkinson's can be countered with exercise, both high intensity and stretch, which maintain function, and prevent progressive decline. A growing body of research shows that exercise promotes neuroplasticity and functional recovery in many neurological disorders.

"The objective was to establish the current evidence for exercise-induced neuroplasticity in people with idiopathic PD, and the results indicate that various forms of physical exercise may lead to changes in a range of markers of neuroplasticity. The narrative synthesis suggests that both brain function and structure can be altered in a positive direction after an exercise period." [1]

Examples of Neuroplasticity

Repetitive movement of a paralysed limb is necessary both in everyday activities and structured workouts to rebuild function. The brain changes and grows when the continuous passage of signals pass through these new pathways many times.

• When someone starts to play a musical instrument, fingers are hesitant whilst learning to place them. To begin with there is a need to practise and repeat and then gradually brain pathways become more diverse and larger. The learner no longer needs to think where to place the fingers. It becomes automatic. The learner moves from conscious incompetence to conscious competence and then unconscious competence when a master pianist can play a complete and complicated musical score without the sheet music.

• Eleanor Maguire of University College London showed in her research that London black cab drivers, who had memorised the names of 25,000 streets and routes to and from different parts of London had enlarged the hippocampal areas of the brain. This area is largely responsible for retained spatial memory. Matched controls of drivers who had not undergone the repetition of memory to remember routes, did not show any difference in size of this brain area. [2]

Use it or Lose it

If a body function is damaged the human reaction may be to stop trying to use that function. If a stroke patient tries to move a damaged arm and finds it doesn't work, he starts using only his non-affected arm. The patient still has the damaged arm but the pathways to and from body to brain will disappear unless messages serving the damaged area are re-started. The implications of this are that in responding to loss of function in the body we need to "use it or lose it" by regular practice. This explains the need for early physiotherapy after most neurological conditions where there is damage to the brain. [See section below: Small Steps Make a Big Difference]

Similar processes of brain re-empowerment occur when the patient's morale improves; and leads to the dedication and drive to do the hard work required within the recovery plan. This needs to be realistic, have fully been discussed with the person concerned and only then fully implemented and repeated with regularity. [See section below: Preparing a Reablement Strategy]

Real-life Experiences

The book *Surviving Stroke* recounts the journey of a consultant neurologist Udo Kischka, supported by his psychologist wife Helen, after a severe stroke until two years after the onset. For example:

"From time to time, he would go barefoot across the bedroom with Helen watching closely, fearful of another fall. At first his big toe had dropped and dragged and seemed to claw the floor as he walked, now there was little, or no drop and the walking movement looked more natural. Again, we have brain plasticity to thank but also ongoing rehab exercises guided by our weekly therapists." [3]

Other accounts of how neuroplasticity can be used constructively and has been harnessed to counter stroke, and other neurological damage, are given in *Stroke Rebel: Optimizing Neuroplasticity to Beat the Odds* by Linda Rådestad and *The Brain's Way of Healing: Remarkable Discoveries from the Frontiers of Neuroplasticity* by Norman Doidge. [4]

"I alleviated chronic pain and became able to walk normally, move my fingers, and even run again. And although it is not perfect at present, I also recovered my ability to speak. All of these things were accomplished AFTER the initial six months. How was I able to recover as well as I have so far, despite all the naysayers? Once I got my overwhelming neuropathic pain under control, I made the conscious decision to ditch my victim mentality forever. Overcoming my pain not only freed up my energy but also taught me the essential lesson that it is possible to rewire my own brain." [Linda Rådestad]

".... it became clear that his claim was not that he had completely cured himself of the disease; rather, as long as he kept up his walking, he could reverse the main movement symptoms of Parkinson's. The changes had so helped him that he was no longer suffering from the main disabilities of PD and was living a full life. [Norman Doidge]

Leading figures in the media and entertainment world give good examples of how the appropriate effort can enable a return to work. Andrew Marr suffered a stroke in 2013 and is now nine years later not only at the top of his profession continuing his media activities but branching out. In 2013 Billy Connolly revealed he was being treated for Parkinson's and only retired from live performances in 2018 but continued to record programmes and make TV appearances and went on to produce his biography.

Small steps leading to improved function need celebrating. A video of before and after the onset showing improved walking, or other important function, boosts morale. Photographs or videos regularly repeated serve as mini-progress reports of recovery – for example, people with neurological conditions regaining the ability to speak, successful career changes, improved mobility. We are reminded that the brain is indeed plastic and that continuing to push on with rehabilitation can lead to very positive changes.

Neuroplasticity and Stroke

When an individual suffers a stroke, a blood clot may form in a blood vessel and causes a blockage of blood flow (ischemic stroke) or a weakened blood vessel burst, causing blood to leak into the brain (haemorrhagic stroke). Decreased blood flow to areas of the brain occurs causing death or damage to neurons. The vital connections between neurons are disrupted.

Connections in different parts of the brain control different functions such as movement, language, speech, and cognition, and the brain adapts better to some areas of damage more than others. Scientists have identified certain areas of the brain that yield neurogenesis (renewed growth).

Understanding the location of your stroke may help you understand the potential effects that may occur. There is no exact answer, but it will give you important insight. For example, a left-brain stroke may cause language difficulties because that's usually where the language centre of the brain resides.

Where a limb is affected the best way to stimulate the brain and activate the neuroplastic response is through repetitive movement. Frequent repetitions of muscle movements or activities, guided by a trained body worker or physiotherapist, will retrain the brain, and cause it to create new neural connections and pathways. The harder a stroke survivor works to retrain the brain, the more likely a positive outcome.

Therapy is designed to enable changes in the properties of existing neural pathways, and the formation of new neural connections. It requires a skilled therapist to determine exactly what needs to be done, how often, and for how long. For example, to recover the use of an arm, it may be necessary to move that arm tens of thousands of times before it begins to generate and use new neural pathways.

The damage inflicted by a stroke is unique to every patient, and so is the recovery process. There are differences in the extent to which individual stroke patients recover. At present some two-thirds will see significant improvements. [5] Great dedication and effort are required.

Significant and lasting improvements won't be achieved in a few days or even a few months.

Stroke Therapies

A leading example of stroke therapy based on neuroplasticity is constraint-induced movement therapy (CIMT). [6]

CIMT involves limiting the movement of the non-affected or stronger arm and instead using the affected or weaker arm more frequently and intensely. For example, by putting the unaffected arm in a sling—while the patient performs various tasks using the affected side. There have been some positive research results with constraint induced therapy; however, it requires much effort and patience from the stroke patient.

CIMT is challenging to stroke patients when they only use their injured side. Many patients understandably feel that the easiest way to resume some type of normality after stroke is to learn how to accomplish daily activities by compensating with their non-impaired side. Not being able to perform tasks like getting dressed, eating, and bathing that they once took for granted is extremely frustrating even though the rationale is clear: The therapy objectives make sense however when the affected person understands the effects of increasing neuroplastic pathways by using the affected side of the body.

Finding the right combination of compensation and task-specific training in stroke survivors is a work-in-progress. But there's an increasing awareness of just how powerful post-stroke CIMT is in reshaping the damaged brain — and that is helping patients move toward better outcomes.

Neuroplasticity, as a natural property of the brain, exists for one's entire life and restorative and rehabilitative interventions can enhance brain repair and stroke recovery even years after stroke onset. [7]

Many of the deficits created by a stroke are treatable through methods that enhance neuroplasticity, including:

Hemiplegia: Hemiplegia occurs when a stroke damages the part of the brain that controls movement on one side of the body. Damage to the left side of the brain causes the right side of the body to react with loss of function including speech difficulties. Therapists have found that active assistive exercise, such as assisting the movement of affected limbs with the unaffected limb, is the best way to treat the lack of mobility.

For example, moving an affected arm or leg with your unaffected hand, or standing, relying on the strength in one leg to compensate for the lack of strength in the other, can stimulate your brain and encourage it to find ways to increase strength and mobility in the weakened limb. The frequency of structured exercise increases the speed and effectiveness of neuroplasticity.

Dysphasia/Aphasia: A right sided stroke can seriously interfere on an individual's ability to communicate, due to damage to the speech centre, resulting in difficulty finding words (dysphasia) or speak at all (aphasia).

There is often, not only impaired speech but also writing, and/or the ability to understand language. The impairment is generally treated through speech therapy, which consists of a series of exercises that stimulate the brain to rewire vital neural connections. Again, there is a direct connection between the frequency of speech therapy and the extent to which speech functions are recovered.

Once a therapy routine is established, supervised by the speech therapist, neuroplasticity is enhanced when the patient works at high intensity with encouragement to do the exercises more frequently. Adding a trained volunteer to support and coach the patient to do the exercises frequently has been found to be most effective compared to a therapist working alone. This combination of trained volunteers working together, following a skilled assessment by a speech therapist, together with frequent repetition and encouragement to repeat, has been shown to be effective. [8]

Speech and language therapy for language impairment is available following brain damage that affects some or all language modalities: expression and understanding of speech, reading, and writing. Approximately one third of people who have a stroke experience aphasia. [9]

Sensory Response: Strokes may also impact an individual's ability to experience sensation in or with their hands, feet, or other parts of the body. Awareness of where limbs are in space – proprioception – may also be affected. (See *A Leg to Stand On* by Oliver Sachs [10] for a graphic account of the effect of its absence.) Generally, impaired sensory response is treated through sensory re-education. This involves exercises that expose the individual to a variety of textures and temperatures. Each exposure to a new sensory experience stimulates the brain and encourages rewiring. Frequent repetition of the same exercises leads to a faster and more complete recovery.

Repetition and Intensity are Vital

Repetitive practice of desired movement patterns helps the brain become stronger by rewiring and reinforcing newly formed neural pathways. Studies in humans and animals have shown that hundreds of repetitions are required per day to elicit change. Anyone that has learned to play the piano can tell you that you must practise every day to get better. The same is true of making changes in the brain after a stroke. This much repetition can seem daunting, but with the help of technology such as rehab-based apps and stroke rehab devices and the help of a carer or family member it becomes easier to fit repetitive movement exercises into a daily routine. [See Appendix 1 – Basic Morning Programme for any Neurological Condition to Prepare for the Day]

Preparing a Reablement Strategy

After the shock of being given the diagnosis of a life changing neurological condition most people will at various times need to come to terms with:

- Denial – "No, not me, it cannot be true"
- Anger – "Why me?"
- Bargaining – attempting to postpone the perceived effect of the diagnosis with "good behaviour"
- Depression – when reacting to their condition, changes in lifestyle and preparing for a perceived lifelong disability
- Acceptance – together with accepting the need to work hard at recovering the best life possible ("what doesn't kill me makes me stronger")

To this end openness about the diagnosis and emphasis on the need to work at recovery is necessary and to keep as mentally and physically fit as possible. Defences come down so that when asked about the illness more open responses occur. Studies show that when people openly share their diagnosis, engagement with rehabilitation improves.

Examples of challenging negative expectations as self-talk are followed by challenge leading to change-talk:

I do not like people asking me about my illness

What is so awful about being asked?

I do not always know what to say

What is so awful about not knowing what to say?

Because I am unsteady on my feet people think I am drunk

What is so awful about them thinking this?

I think they are laughing at me

What is it so awful about them laughing at you?

I do not think they will take me seriously.

What is so awful about not being taken seriously?

It means they do not believe me.

What is so awful if they do not believe you?

I feel they do not see me for who I am.

How can they see you as you are if you do not tell them about your illness? They will see me recover as neuroplasticity rebuilds my ability to function again.

Overwhelmed at Diagnosis?

The way the brain works means that every time you feel out of control and overwhelmed about the things you "must do", you get better at feeling overwhelmed. Every time you get frustrated about being unwell, you get better at being frustrated. Is it surprising that 60% of people with PD become depressed over the lifetime of living with PD?

By now you will understand that it is not surprising that fear and anxiety about having a diagnosis that implies continuing loss of function, activates the Fight, Flight or Fold stress response.

For example, you decide to meet a friend for lunch. Without even thinking about it, you start to feel anxious. When you are faced with this situation, your brain searches your memory files to find out how to respond to this kind of situation. The brain has associated meeting a friend with anxiety. As this has happened several times, the brain starts telling the body that this is an appropriate time to start to feel anxious even though this is unhelpful. The brain thinks that you are under threat, and you start to activate the fight, flight, or fold response. The threat response, when activated, stops you doing what you need to do, and you stay in and get more depressed and anxious.

Living with PD is helped greatly by two methods called cognitive behavioural therapy and mindfulness.

Mindfulness

- An approach that helps the individual regain present moment awareness, and away from anxious thoughts and feelings: particularly when you catastrophise your present situation, and this has become an unhelpful pattern.

- The individual is then taught to use mindfulness approaches that bring you back to being present in the moment. [11]

- To bring us back to being present in the present moment breathing techniques are an important link between mind and body.

- To induce calm, you learn to engage the "quieting and calming capacity" of the brain. You can re-balance and calm your excitable brain by changing breathing patterns. The in breath is shortened and the outbreath lengthened. [12] This can lead to the ability to counterbalance the sympathetic action orientated response – linked to the in breath with the calm parasympathetic rest and relax response (linked to the outbreath), where clarity of thinking is enhanced. [13]

- You now know the effect of too much challenge, leading to excessive and sustained stress, on your inner physiology, and so it will be no surprise to you that this can result in you feeling exhausted. 50% of people with PD are tired most of the time. With conscious mindfulness and awareness, you can change this response so that we do not feel anxious and stressed because you know the signals and can respond appropriately [14]. For a fuller explanation see the book *Emotional Healing* [15]

Cognitive behavioural Therapy or Coaching

- A counselling method used frequently in the NHS to help you to change negative thoughts and deal more effectively with problems in your life by changing your thoughts and unwanted emotions. [16]

Small Steps Make a Big Difference

When a person has had a stroke, new skills need to be learnt and practised many times a day for neuroplasticity to occur to aid greater independence in functioning. This is made easier by getting the person to use their mind, e.g. saying what they are going to do in the first person singular – they themselves are initiating the movement by saying "I clasp my hands together". [17] This is the basis of the Conductive Education approach.

The normal person has no awareness of how they are using their body, they only know what they want to do [18], e.g. make a cup of tea. So, they have no awareness of what the body needs to do to achieve this aim. If a person becomes disabled then they will need to learn how to achieve their functional aims, such as moving in bed to get comfortable, or how to get out of bed in the most normal way moving towards their affected side to increase weightbearing and so stimulate the weaker muscles.

Conductive Education uses a cognitive approach where the programme is divided into a collection of tasks and each in turn is broken down into task parts where the conductor says the action, the patient/participant repeats the action in the first person singular and then carries out the action to counting, known as rhythmical intention. This help the person to concentrate, remember and repeat the action correctly many times until the repetition of the words is no longer needed showing that they are relearning a skill. Here movement, function and speech are used together. Since the programme of a group session usually takes place in lying, sitting, standing and walking all parts of the body are involved. [19] [Appendix 5 illustrates this and shows how an affected hand can be brought back into use.]

A Lying Programme

A lying programme can give a disabled person confidence in moving and changing position in bed which is a preparation for them moving from lying into sitting over the affected side. An example of a lying programme – a series of movements and exercises while lying in bed and not having to worry about balance – to help improve independence and maintain abilities is given in Appendix 1 – Basic Morning Programme to Prepare for the Day. Its value is explained both from a physiotherapy and a physiological viewpoint. It would need to be approached according to the individual person.

Good Positioning

The person needs to relearn how to function efficiently which is linked to relearning how to use their body well and how to relax normally as they would if they did not have a neurological disorder. For example, if the person with a stroke does not support the elbow or the hand in a natural way, this will lead to pain and stiffness in the shoulder and the arm. This is important also from the perspective of being accepted into society by not looking abnormal which puts up a barrier that need not be there. [See Appendix 2 – Normal Positions to Support Muscles & Joints, for examples of different positions that a person will take up unconsciously] These positions/postures have a role in putting the body in positions to stretch or weightbear the limbs, hands and feet

Learning to Walk

Relearning how to walk after a stroke can be addressed by using a ladder chair. Here the whole body is involved as is normal. [See Appendix 3 – Use of a Ladder Chair] The person stands in front of the back of a ladder chair whose four legs form a stable base. Immediately the person has a visual template of symmetry which is needed for good balance. The person is then taught to clasp their hands and then guided to put the weaker hand onto the appropriate rung of the ladder back at the correct height. The stronger hand can keep the weaker hand in place. The instruction can be given by using the personal pronoun so that the person is learning to help and guide him/herself. This also helps memory, concentration, and the body to open new pathways or stimulate dormant cells taking advantage of inherent neuroplasticity.

By pushing the chair forwards this encourages arm and wrist extension through weightbearing on the rung with a forward movement of the arms, away from the spastic pattern. Through speech and counting a natural rhythm can be encouraged to work on extension of the hip with good alternate weightbearing on the feet.

With repetition and practice, walking can progress to walking with a stick with a small base. Simultaneously work will continue in lying and sitting, where the person will practise going from sitting to standing with hands clasped, arms in extension to work on strengthening the legs for weightbearing and equal balance. Then work can be carried out in the kitchen or bathroom so that the person can use time well, e.g. while waiting for the kettle to boil, sideways walking can be practised which is always useful in a kitchen. In a supermarket the person can be encouraged to push the trolley with both hands as practised with the ladder chair.

REFERENCES

[1] Hanna Johansson, Maria Hagstromer, Wilhelmus J. A. Grooten, Erika Franzen, *Exercise-Induced Neuroplasticity in Parkinson's Disease: A Metasynthesis of the Literature,* Neural Plasticity, Vol. 2020, Article ID 8961493 https://pubmed.ncbi.nlm.nih.gov/32256559/

[2] Eleanor A. Maguire, Katherine Woollett, Hugo J. Spiers, *London taxi drivers and bus drivers: a structural MRI and neuropsychological analysis,* Hippocampus, 2006, 16(12):1091-101 https://pubmed.ncbi.nlm.nih.gov/17024677/

[3] Helen Kennerly, Udo Kischka, *Surviving Stroke,* Robinson, 2020

[4] Linda Rådestad, *Stroke Rebel: Optimizing Neuroplasticity to Beat the Odds,* Brain Rehab Distribution, October 2019

Norman Doidge, *The Brain's Way of Healing: Remarkable Discoveries from the Frontiers of Neuroplasticity,* Penguin Books, 2016

[5] Moheb Costandi, *Neuroplasticity (The MIT Press Essential Knowledge Series),* The MIT Press, 2016

[6] David J. Lin, Seth P. Finklestein, Steven C. Cramer, *New directions in treatments targeting stroke recovery,* Stroke, December 2018, 49(12): 3107–3114 https://pubmed.ncbi.nlm.nih.gov/30571435/

[7] Li-Ru Zhaoa, Alison Willing, *Enhancing endogenous capacity to repair a stroke-damaged brain: An evolving field for stroke research,* Progress in Neurobiology, Vol. 163–164, April–May 2018, pp5-26 https://pubmed.ncbi.nlm.nih.gov/29476785/

[8] Peter Langhorne, Julie Bernhardt, Gert Kwakkel, *Stroke Rehabilitation,* Lancet, 2011 May 14; 377(9778): 1693-702 https://pubmed.ncbi.nlm.nih.gov/21571152/

[9] Marian C. Brady, Helen Kelly, Jon Godwin, Pam Enderby, Pauline Campbell, *Speech and language therapy for aphasia following stroke,* Cochrane Database of Systematic Reviews, June 2016 https://pubmed.ncbi.nlm.nih.gov/27245310/

[10] Oliver Sacks, *A Leg to Stand On,* Duckworth, 1998

[11] *The neuroscience behind mindfulness*, Harvard Neuro Blog https://harvardneuro.wordpress.com/2016/01/06/the-neuroscience-behind-mindfulness/

[12] David Beales and colleagues, *Chapter on Breath, Reclaim Health*, Amazon, 2020

[13] Ellen J. Langer, *Mindfulness*, Da Capo Lifelong Books, 2020 revised

[14] Julie Corliss, *Six relaxation techniques to reduce stress*, Harvard Heart Letter https://www.health.harvard.edu/mind-and-mood/six-relaxation-techniques-to-reduce-stress

[15] David Beales, Helen Whitten, *Chapter 2, Emotional Healing*, Wiley, 2010

[16] Helen Whitten, *Cognitive Behavioural Coaching*, Wiley, 2009

[17] Stephen J. Page, Peter Levine, Anthony Leonard, *Mental Practice in Chronic Stroke – Results of a Randomized, Placebo-Controlled Trial*, Stroke, 2007, 38:1293–1297 https://www.ahajournals.org/doi/full/10.1161/01.STR.0000260205.67348.2b

[18] N. A. Bernstein, *The co-ordination and regulation of movements*, Pergamon Press, 1967

[19] Roberta O'Shea, Mary Jones, Katie Lightfoot, *Examining Conductive Education: Linking Science, Theory, and Intervention*, Archives of Rehabilitation Research and Clinical Translation, Vol. 2, Issue 4, December 2020, 100077

~~~~~
~~~~~

Chapter 7
What it Means to be a Carer

Sara Challice

A Bit of My Story

I had only been seeing my boyfriend for six weeks when he was diagnosed with a brain tumour. At the time, I remember saying to him, "Just get better Neal, I'm here for you".

I meant well but had no idea of the detrimental effects caring for him would end up having on my own health.

Neal had a long operation, six weeks of radiotherapy and six months of chemotherapy. During this time, I had moved into his home to be with him, driving him to and from hospital, looking after him, whilst I continued to work full time.

Working and caring was full on and a juggling act, but after those six months, Neal was given the all clear by his neurosurgeon and was told he was disease-free. This was such a relief. We could now get on with our lives. The following Christmas Neal proposed to me, but only a few weeks after our engagement, he started having the same side-effects which had led him to his diagnosis – pins and needles down one side of his body. This tell-tale sign and hunch was right. The brain tumour had returned but this time it was inoperable.

Neal realised what this would mean to me – being wed to a man with brain cancer, and said that I didn't have to marry him. But I refused to allow cancer to dictate our lives. We were on this journey together and we were in love. So, we brought the wedding forward and saw it as a huge celebration with all our friends and family, however long we had.

But five more years of chemotherapy resumed, Neal was having falls as his mobility continued to decline, and I left my job and career in the city to care for him full-time. I also wanted to spend quality time with him as I knew his time was limited.

Neal was frequently in and out of hospital, and they gave him six weeks of physiotherapy when he had come home. This was wonderful as the physiotherapist would visit him at home. But after the six weeks, the physiotherapy was stopped, but Neal's decline did not – as with most with neurological conditions. Even though he was exercising, Neal had more falls and more trips to hospital. When I rang the physiotherapist to ask for more help for Neal, I was bluntly told that they had closed his file and we had to go back to the GP to get a further referral.

I was shocked at their response. Neal fell many times, and as he was 17 stone and almost twice my size and weight, I was left struggling to care for him. I emailed the physiotherapist and said how uncaring I had found their response. Even though they had closed Neal's file, he clearly still needed regular physiotherapy to help to him remain safe in the home.

Then one afternoon, a MacMillan nurse visited us, and as we sat chatting in our living room, she told us of INS, a neuro charity based in Twickenham which gave one-to-one physiotherapy. "Really?", I asked.

It sounded too good to be true! Both Neal and myself then went to a talk by Sir Ranulph Fiennes – an INS event to raise funds and awareness for the charity and the great work they do. This is where I met Ellie Kinnear – the founder of INS, the CEO and a number of wonderful people involved with the charity.

Neal was then registered with INS and started to have one-to-one physiotherapy at their centre in Twickenham. I was also supported as a carer. The wonderful thing about INS is that they do not close your file. It remains open for as long as needed, which is certainly more caring and more supportive within our community.

A few years later, Neal had a stroke and ended up in a hospital bed in our living room, with a PEG feeding tube and unable to speak. With the help of paid carers, we hoisted him out of bed each day and into his wheelchair. A tragic fate for Neal, but what about the carer?

For me, caring became nursing care. It was 24/7and relentless. My whole world revolved around attempting to keep my husband alive. At night I would also have a baby monitor on upstairs, just in case Neal had one of his choking fits – a regular occurrence. At some point during the night, I would throw myself down the stairs and tend to him. For years I slept with one ear open.

Family and friends would ask how Neal was, but what about the carer? I was constantly in response mode, ensuring he had what he needed, and my world became a much smaller place. For one whole year, I didn't even head back to see my parents or family. It wasn't until my grandfather died suddenly that I realised I had put all my love into one person and left the rest of my family to one side. I recognised this needed to change – I needed to see my family.

I also saw myself as responsible for Neal's life – a tall order when looking after a loved one who is palliative care and could be gone at any time… for years. I would describe caring for a husband with a brain tumour like this; although it was Neal who had the brain tumour, I woke up brain cancer every day for 13 years. It may not have been physically in my head, but it affected every area of my life until it made me both mentally and physically ill.

I was also grieving. Grieving for the loss of what we had already lost. Just to be able to have a conversation and go out for a meal was a thing of the past. I was also grieving for the impending loss of my husband – I knew it was only a matter of time.

If I did manage to get out and see friends and have a break, I felt guilty in leaving him with a paid carer. I even turned down respite, feeling guilty leaving Neal in a hospice whilst I had a week's holiday break. It wasn't until I finally fell ill and desperately asked for a week's respite at our local hospice, that the head nurse, Julia, told me that carers need regular breaks. It's too late when you have fallen ill.

I finally managed to get away, to a silent retreat of all things! It was in this place, having peace and recuperation that I realised I hadn't just left myself last on the list, I wasn't even on the list! And because I wanted to look like I was coping and didn't want to appear a failure to friends and family. I had put on a brave face, always smiling, when in fact I was treading water and slowly sinking.

At this time I realised I needed to make changes to ensure that not only did I survive caring for Neal, but actually find ways to enjoy life again – guilt free! These days, weeks and months wouldn't be here again – this was my life too.

Life is not about abstaining and enduring, it is still about enjoying, especially if you are a carer.

Three in five of us will be a carer at some point in our lifetime, and with an ageing population and more of us surviving critical illness, many more of us will need care within our homes – which will often falling on to other family members.

Sadly, around 70% of carers fall ill from the stress and burden of caring. There clearly needs to be more done to support those caring for loved ones. I also know of a number of carers who are now long-term sick, they believe, due to the stress of caring for many years. Tara cared for her husband for many years, as he deteriorated due to the brain tumour. Only eight weeks after he had passed, Tara was diagnosed with multiple sclerosis. She is now in a wheelchair and their son, in his 20s, who should be out making the most of his life, is now caring for her. It is like a ripple effect of stress and illness running through the family.

Carers clearly need more support from the government and within the community – and charities like INS can offer wonderful support. In my last year of caring I started to write, *Who Cares? – How to care for yourself whilst caring for a loved one*, which is available on Amazon. Here are 10 tips to help empower carers to look after their health and well-being, whilst becoming more resilient:

Top Tips for Carers

1. Check in with yourself

As a carer, you're often too busy being there for everyone else that you ignore your own health. You may even be suppressing your emotions, whilst feeling that you're coping, but in fact you may be treading water, and slowly sinking. The pressure can build up, bit by bit, and go unnoticed. It's best to not wait until a crisis strikes but to keep an eye on your own health, as difficult as this can be at times.

Do you have a good friend or family member you could check in with for a short time, once a week? This can be either face-to-face (socially distancing), over the phone or via skype. Or you could try journaling. Writing down how you're feeling and the issues you're experiencing can help you to observe what's actually happening. This can help lead to making better choices to give yourself space to be there for you.

2. Put the feelers out

There are so many great charities and services available, but often we have no idea they are actually there. Have you called your local carers centre lately? Even though their doors may be closed for now, they may still be tirelessly working, calling around and offering lots of support.

They may also have suggestions of other services in your local area which may be of great benefit.

3. Accept where you are now

When we start caring, we may notice many changes happening around us. Firstly, your loved one's health may have altered, and what you now have to do on a daily basis may have changed significantly. Also, you may have had to give up work to care, and even if not, your own world may have become smaller as you focus on another. Change is an inevitable part to life and resisting what we cannot change will only increase our frustration. So instead, look for what you can change.

4. Rise to the challenge

Caring can bring up many issues, some you would never have even thought of! As challenges strike, we have a choice in how we react. We can either play the victim role or we can ask ourselves, what do I need to do differently here? What am I learning from this? Because challenges are here to help us grow. Remember, there is only so much you can do for loved ones, but you also need to be there for you. Ensure your boundaries, to look after your own health and well-being.

5. Drop the mask and ask

You may be putting on a brave face, as you feel you need to be strong for loved ones. You may also accept your situation and feel you have to struggle on alone, hiding your feelings, for fear of being judged. If others ask how you are, be honest, open up and ask for more support. Otherwise, if they are not aware, how will they know you need help? Also, you never know what they might offer. If you do ask family for help, try getting a date in the diary to make the commitment more certain. Otherwise, time may drift along with empty promises. And if they do offer help, let them know how appreciative you are. This may help inspire them to do more!

6. Surround yourself with those who care

Your Ultimate Support Network is key and not everyone will have the love and compassion you need right now. Who lifts you up when you are feeling down? Who puts a smile on your face? Although we are physically distancing to stay safe and protect ourselves and vulnerable loved ones, we can still socially connect by phone, Zoom or Skype. If others have not been in touch for some time, it may be good to be the instigator and call them instead. You could write a list of those who always cheer you up, and take a short time each day to get in touch with them. I have a great chapter in my book called "Taps & Drains", which goes into more detail on this, and was very much my 'A-ha' moment whilst caring!

7. Be kind to yourself

We are often there for others but forget to be there for ourselves. Caring is hard enough, but often we may criticise and judge ourselves, beating ourselves up. No wonder so many of us are prone to falling ill!

Be kind to yourself and be there for you. Be your own best friend. What do you need right now to make you feel better? Give yourself permission each day to do at least one thing for yourself, because these days, weeks and months won't be back and you deserve to enjoy your life, as difficult as life may be.

8. Take a break

We all need to recharge our batteries, and have time out, but often you may feel guilty heading out to enjoy yourself when a loved one is left at home. Even so, you still need regular breaks, not only to recoup, but also to enjoy quality time. You're not just here for a loved one, you are also here for you! In having a break, you will then be in a better frame of mind and more able to deal with the challenges. I would find, that in going into the outside space, helped me reflect on the inside space. So, instead of seeing each day as a list of chores, try taking a short break between each one. This will help you pace the day, otherwise if you just do this and just do that, you'll just fall into bed exhausted at the end of the day!

9. Focus on the good stuff

Carers are often in survival mode, wanting to make sure everything and everyone is okay, but continually focussing on the problems and issues, can lead to us forgetting about all the great things that are in our lives. This can easily become a pattern of behaviour. One way to stop negative thoughts is to pop an elastic band around your wrist. The next time you notice yourself starting to have a particular negative thought, give it a quick ping to stop yourself. If I was having a challenging day, I would think of five things I was grateful for – maybe a hot shower that morning or my comfy bed last night. As soon as I started appreciating the little things, I would begin to feel better, shifting my mood.

10. You are amazing!

If you are a carer, you are amazing! Continuing to care for a loved one shows real dedication, strength and resilience. Not everybody can do what you do. Giving up your time, energy and life to be there for another is without doubt an inspiring and selfless act and it's not easy. When other carers share their life stories, I often tell them how humbled I feel. Although they often say they don't feel like they are doing anything particularly special, they are, and so are you!

The True Value of Care

In the last year of caring for Neal, I remember my mum saying, "I never thought my daughter would be a carer!"

I knew exactly what she meant. When it comes to our hopes and dreams for ourselves and for others, caring for a loved one for years is not usually what we have in mind! But caring for a loved one is so much more than we often perceive.

I gave a talk at the Houses of Parliament a number of years ago entitled, "A decade of caring." Straight after I had spoken, a neurosurgeon got up to speak. He said he was often asked what was the best criteria for surviving a brain tumour. I stood pondering and thinking it must be the latest chemotherapy or radiotherapy treatment, but his answer surprised us all. He said the best criteria for surviving a brain tumour was actually marital status. I loved his insight! Personally, I don't think you need to be married, because if you are the one who has fallen seriously ill and you have somebody fighting your corner and being an emotional and physical rock for you – this is a huge boost. Not only that, you still have a reason to live – the love of another.

I believe my love and care for Neal kept him alive for years longer. I remember after he had been in the hospice for a week, to give me a break, that he went downhill rapidly. But when I got him home again, he visibly improved within days. Love and care keep others alive. We need to value carers and all that they do behind closed doors, often for many years. It is estimated that unpaid carers save the UK economy £132 billion a year – this is the same cost of the second NHS. Amazing! – but not when so many of us end up paying with our own health. We need to value and support our carers and recognise the value of good care – both in perception and in monetary terms. You just never know, one day it maybe you needing care.

~~~~~
~~~~~

Chapter 8
Addressing Issues

Parkinson's - The Four Pillars

Alexander Reed. Alexander has lived with Parkinson's for over 15 years. He is director of the European Parkinson Therapy Centre. www.parkinsontherapy.com

~~~~~

We all have a degenerative condition in us called ageing, yet most people of 70 years do not blame their age for their reduced ability to do things, indeed we normally celebrate our birthday!!! When we have Parkinson's, this accepting and adapting to this reality is harder, as we are less prepared for it (it was never part of the "plan"). But nevertheless, we must adapt, and as with old age, accept that we are simply less able.

Our health services in Europe are also not always in our favour. We get the diagnosis, a packet of pills and an appointment somewhere down the line. It comes as a shock to the system and it is little understood that it is a shock to the whole family, too. What are we meant to do? What is going to happen?

Parkinson's affects the whole family, and the whole family needs support and reassurance.

It's not surprising that over 50% of people with Parkinson's are clinically depressed, and that the vast majority do not seek help, but head for the nearest desk and hide under it, figuratively speaking! The sad truth about Parkinson's is that the real truth is never made clear.

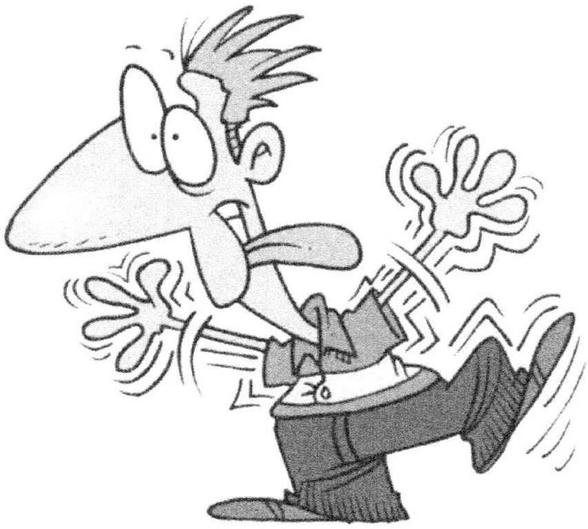

I wish that when first diagnosed I had been told; "You can reduce symptoms by up to 40%; you can help slow progression, and your life will become more precious, not less, if you make the right choices."

Some of us are reluctant to admit that we have Parkinson's, almost as if we are afraid to be looked upon as different or weaker. Yet even the person who comes last in an event in the
~~~~~

Paralympics is applauded, because he or she has chosen to fight. Anybody who faces adversity with determination is stronger for it.

Words like "Parkinson's made me a better man" or "Parkinson's was an opportunity" make little sense at that moment of diagnosis but are often used by those who learn to take control

According to one famous study (Parkinson's Outcomes Project), the number one thing that destroys the quality of life of a person with Parkinson's is fear, anxiety, apathy and depression, NOT Parkinson's but our reaction and emotional state. This point is essential in learning to live with Parkinson's.

Time and time again, I meet families devastated by Parkinson's, and week in and week out we explain that Parkinson's may bring a change of life, but sometimes that change can actually strengthen the family and be a new opportunity for your life. Parkinson's does not destroy our lives; it just means we must adapt to the limits it imposes.

Our therapy model is based on the concept that there are four key elements (what we call "Pillars") to maintain quality of life. Medicines are of course at the core, but like a house with one wall, it will not keep the roof up. Medicines to a depressed person will not change his or her life. You need all four Pillars delivered in one place intensively.

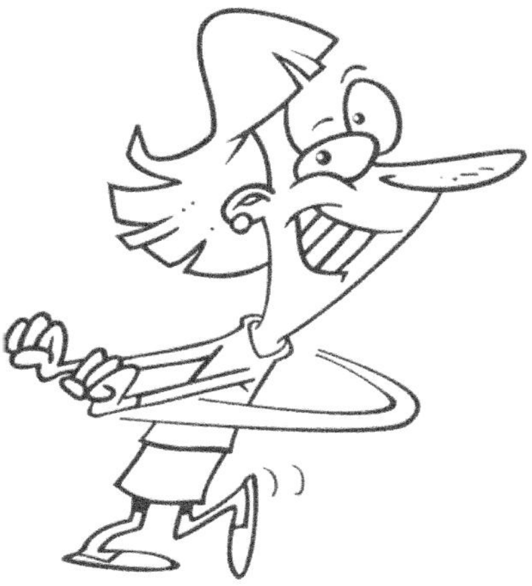

If you want to learn a foreign language, one hour per week will not work. Two weeks of full-immersion will have a much higher impact - and even more so if you apply what you have learned and speak that language every day for the rest of your life. It is the same for Parkinson's, an appointment here and a dance class there will not be enough to change our quality of life.

So, what are the four Pillars of Parkinson's?

First Pillar - Medicine

Medicine, as we previously mentioned, is what keeps us moving and eases some aspects of Parkinson's. One well-known British neurologist told me recently, *"We know a lot about Parkinson's, but we don't and can't know what is truly like to have Parkinson's"*. This is a remarkable insight, and probably why this neurologist is so exceptional. I have seen many people who have visited over 10 different neurologists and complain that they have not found the right one who can "solve" their problems. It is unrealistic that in a 20-minute appointment a neurologist can solve all the complex issues surrounding Parkinson's with a pill. Medicine is an essential pillar not a crutch.

In the coming years there will be medicines that actually stop or reverse (not cure) our Parkinson's, but embarrassingly today the frontline drug DOES NOT improve or stop Parkinson's, it helps us to move. It was discovered in 1910 (!) Incredible but true.

Second Pillar - Physical Movement

Physical movement is now understood better. Like taking pills, it is now scientifically accepted that it must be done daily to see and maintain results. Regularity is better than quantity. But what must we do to improve our condition with movement? Walking is a basic and fundamental aspect of daily life with Parkinson's. It produces a neuroprotective effect; in short, it helps slow down neurodegeneration, which is good for everybody, but especially for those of us with Parkinson's.

Tango therapy, going to the gym and physiotherapy are often mentioned, but in reality, if not done regularly, they have limited effects and are not specific to you. Individual therapy will get results

Studies show that physiotherapy needs to be combined with conscious thought: "Think before you move." This point is often missed and is based on the concept of neuroplasticity. If someone breaks a leg, they may do physiotherapy, but for us the problem is inside our head, so physiotherapy must be combined with conscious thought. If we think and correct our posture, length of stride and arm movement, and then actually consciously keep doing it, we find that over a short period of time the brain adapts and this correction becomes automatic. Rather like if you always sleep on your side, and one day, because you have a broken rib, you are forced to sleep on our back. For the first few nights this probably means little sleep, but then our brain accepts the new reality, and even after the rib is healed, you continue to sleep happily on your back.

Group therapy is popular too, but everybody is different in his or her Parkinson's. Take four chefs and give them the same ten ingredients, and you'll end up with four different meals. If you really want to reduce your symptoms, you need to work individually with a neurophysio specialist to identify, correct and learn to maintain this correction.

Pillar 3 - Lifestyle

Lifestyle is perhaps the least understood, and hence the less treated of the four Pillars. Apart from well-known points about what and when we eat and the avoidance of stress, what is essential to understand is that we have a CHOICE in how we live our lives. We can choose to be apathetic and negative, or we can choose to take control. We can choose to delegate our quality of life to a neurologist or to our spouses, or we can choose to focus our lives on doing what we can enjoy. Choosing to continue at full speed is not a choice; it is denial. Full speed is like driving a car fast with an engine that is slowly losing power; at some stage it will break down. Life will change, but who says we cannot decide how it should change? If we choose to do less but do more of what we enjoy, then our quality of life is maintained.

Pillar 4 - Psychology

We use the ACMA approach. The first step is to ACCEPT we have Parkinson's; that means accepting something we don't want, but just like ageing, it is a fact. How can we fight something if we do not accept it exists? Like going into a boxing ring with a blindfold, we are going to get hit hard. Take the blindfold off, and we can hit back! COMPREHENSION of the reality of Parkinson's makes us stronger, as we realise we can influence progression and symptoms. It's much harder to fight in a war we do not believe in or a war in which we don't understand the strategy. Only if we accept and comprehend it can we be MOTIVATED as we see the positive effects of taking control, and this will only be effective if we combine what we need to do with what we enjoy doing. We cannot stay motivated if we are always doing things we have to do with no reward. Dopamine is released into our brain when we do something enjoyable, so we become more inclined to take a long, healthy walk if, for instance, it brings us a reward like a stop at an ice cream shop or your local pub.

These three stages bring about real ACTION, which we can sustain and believe in. Too many people talk about what we must do (the action), without having accepted, understood and decided to actually do it.

How we perceive our Parkinson's has a real impact on how we live with our Parkinson's.

If one of the above Pillars goes down, it may pull down the others too! That's why apathy and depression are so destructive. If we stop caring, we stop exercising and we stop living. We are then left with just the medicines – back to square one – and worse, we enter what one leading neurologist called "The Vortex of Apathy". The vortex pulls us down, eliminates neuroprotection and neuroplasticity, and it destroys people with Parkinson's and the lives of those around them.

Looking back at what we were able to do before Parkinson's instead of all the things we can still do is at the root of many people's depression. Looking forward, we may experience fear and anxiety. "Where will I be in ten years? What does the future hold?" WRONG question, nobody can see the future. All of this put together can create the apathy so associated with Parkinson's. The truth is that neither looking backwards or forwards is relevant. It is today that is relevant, and we should focus on managing and maximizing our lives every day: seeing the funny side, learning the truth and living a full life with Parkinson's.

~~~~~

Unexplained Symptoms

David Beales

~~~~~

Medicine must harness mind body interactions - You were wise to select Descartes' dualism - separating mind from body - as the topic for your leading letter. [Letter in the Financial Times, 26 February 2022]

This 17th century model does indeed still drive modern medicine as illustrated by separate hospital dealing with physical and mental illnesses and it needs much more analysis. In addition to placebo studies research in both neuroscience and continuity of care reveals strong mind body interactions.'

In Britain the role of general practise doctors as the medical specialty accepting both patients physical and emotional problems and treating both, needs re-evaluation. [Denis Pereira - Former Chairman Academy of Medical Royal Colleges Devon, UK. Letter in the Financial Times, 5-6 March 2022]

Many symptoms such as those following a diagnosis of a neurological condition are brought about by mechanisms that are not due to the condition itself. [1]

Many symptoms in the section below, despite conventional medical investigation remain unexplained. The predicament of the person with a neurological condition has not been understood within a whole person context. The distress leads to a continued reaction of distress and occurs when essential human needs are not being met. Symptoms which signal this are:

Chest Pain; Feeling tense; Blurred vision; Dizzy spells; Feeling confused (brain fog); Faster or deeper breathing; Feeling short of breath; Tight feelings in the chest; Boated feelings in the stomach; Tingling fingers; Unable to breathe deeply; Stiff fingers or arms; Tight feelings around the mouth; Cold hands and feet; Heart racing and/or palpitations; Feelings of anxiety.

When scored as a questionnaire for each symptom as: 0 never; 1 rarely; 2 sometimes; 3 often; 4 very often, the maximum score is 64.

Scores over 23 suggest that the life situation of the individual has led to excessive anxiety and over breathing. Attention to reversing the abnormal breathing pattern with counselling to identify and lower excessive life stress and too much physical and mental load, with attention to unmet need is likely to be helpful.

These essential needs include enough Attention, Purpose and Goals, Connection to others, Creativity and Stimulation, being understood, a sense of being enough in Control.

In Parkinson's the loss of dopamine producing neurological cells affects movement, bladder and bowel function, fatigue, anxiety, and depression, and often brings with it chronic stress. The individual moves beyond their perceived limit of tolerance for the situation they find themselves facing.

This results in the fight, flight or freeze mechanisms within the body-mind to flood the individual with stress hormones designed by evolution to deal with the threatening situation. [2] Unless we understand these mechanisms and deal with them by switching on calm, purposeful, actions with good thinking strategies we are likely to stay stressed and this in turn can aggravate the neurological symptoms.

We also know that 50 per cent of symptoms presenting to GP's and medical syndromes, such as irritable bowel syndrome, have no medically identifiable cause. Patients with so-called medically unexplained symptoms take up a large proportion of GPs' consultation time, returning to the surgery again and again, and that of specialists in a variety of hospital departments such as gastroenterology, gynaecology, rheumatology, cardiology, neurology, and dentistry. [3] [4] [5]

People commonly develop physical symptoms when they are in a state of heightened anxiety and are at the limit of their tolerance. The physiological changes are measurable and the drive system with not enough rest and recovery is switched on. [6]

Not relating the two, they are anxious to find the physical cause. Indeed, many of both doctors and patients think that such an approach is all that is required. If, after doing the conventional tests, doctors simply say that they can find no cause for the symptoms and attempt merely to offer reassurance without working with patients to understand what is going on, satisfaction with the consultation is likely to be poor and trust diminished. [7]

People often feel angry and rejected if told nothing is wrong, "it's just the Parkinson's", when clearly something else is wrong, other than Parkinson's. The good news is that many of these symptoms can be understood and helped to go on their way.

How do we break out of that cycle?

The Physiological Facts

When lives become over-pressured or impoverished, because of excessive emotional arousal or pressures from the outer world, such as dealing with a neurological condition, work or relationship difficulties, the internal systems protest.

What happens to us in such situations can be clearly understood in physiological terms. Homeostasis, or the maintenance of self-regulation, is the basis of health. When disturbed, mind–body protest is the result.

There is a complex inter-relationship between messenger hormones of emotion, [8] and the autonomic nervous system – the part of the nervous system responsible for control of bodily functions that are not under conscious direction. [9]

These systems in turn interplay with the immune system, which is intimately connected with our mind–body state. [10]

The body, in adapting to evolutionary challenges, has developed an array of responses that maintain the constancy of its internal state and resist harmful imbalances. A thirst reaction protects us from dehydration, for instance. Tiredness and fatigue are responses that serve to warn us to stop before we become exhausted. However, the ever-changing pressures in our complex lives can lead us to ignore or overrule these sensations. Asking yourself a question when troubled by unexplained symptoms such as "my symptoms are with me in order to tell me to stop doing X------------; and start Y------------"

The Human Function Curve

To explain the difference between healthy arousal and exhausted over-arousal, cardiologist Peter Nixon developed the human function curve. [11]

Healthy functioning and healthy fatigue, on the up slope of the curve, are experienced when we are coping well, adapting to changes in our lives or making supreme efforts that have successful outcomes. Exhaustion and ill health on the down slope, often followed by breakdown, occur when we are not coping and adapting effectively and we feel defeated, no matter what efforts we make to deal with the demands in our lives.

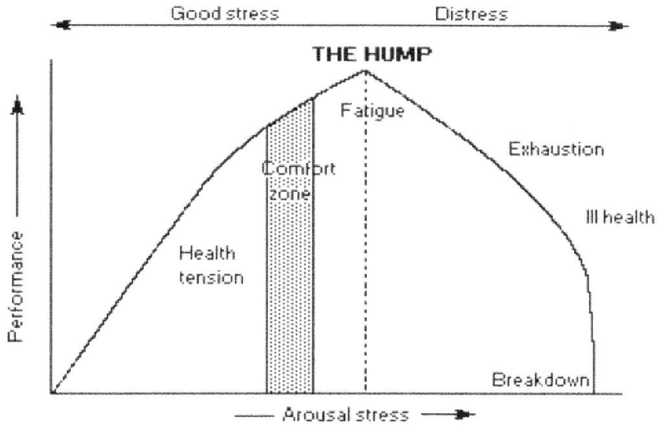

Adapted from: Nixon, P: Practioner, 1979.

Too much sustained, unhealthy, down slope arousal leads to the loss of internal balance and results in reduced performance and a mind–body system in overdrive. In this state, the metabolism is struggling and cholesterol, blood sugar and blood pressure are often raised, resulting in ill health.

The more aroused we become, the more sleep, which would be to some degree restorative, decreases. Signals of mind–body protest multiply. For instance, sufferers from irritable bowel syndrome may also commonly experience back pain, fatigue and loss of libido. Negative emotions, such as frustration and despair, can trigger exhaustion, which in turn can trigger breathing pattern disorders, because of the perceived threat to survival eliciting fight, flight or freeze reactions. [12]

Providing Patients with Physiological and Physical Explanations

It is always important to remember that symptoms that are developing side by side with a neurological condition may be initially unexplained. They do sometimes result from added pathology, but GPs' training is in the early recognition of pathological disease and their medical vigilance is always required.

There are several ways to give physical evidence of imbalance in a patient's body system and that they are stuck in a state of sustained arousal. For example, breathing chemistry is an indicator and can be analysed, a saliva swab can show raised levels of the stress hormone cortisol, and a sensor on the skin can pick up heart rate variability.

Creating Solutions

The right approach allows individuals to understand their symptoms in the context of their predicament and makes patients more likely to work with their medical adviser to return to a state of healthy functioning and well-being.

They accept the term "functional disturbance", whereas they reject terms such as "medically unexplained symptoms" or a psychological explanation, and rightly so. [13]

Nutrition

Nutrition is very important. As mentioned, an over-pressured state of internal arousal results in raised cholesterol, raised blood sugar, raised cortisol levels, and disturbed immune function.

In such a state, the individual is likely not to have paid attention to good nutrition and may often have tried to drive a malfunctioning and exhausted mind and body with the help of excessive alcohol, comfort foods or stimulants. The microbiome-the different bacteria in the gut-is thought to be abnormal in PD.

Choices that restore good nutrition, initially supported by supplementation, including re-balancing neuronal circuitry with omega-three fatty acids and micronutrients, are often useful supportive adjuncts.

A Calm Environment

If, according to their own account, someone's energy is well down the human function curve, it is often advisable, if it is possible, to withdraw from the situation in which the symptoms arose to a place where recovery can occur.

In Ancient Greece, over-pressured patricians withdrew into healing temples, where they were allowed rest, sleep and recover. Body work, including massage, hot baths combined with music and a calming environment, made up the initial first stage of healing. Only later were exercise, reflection and reasoning encouraged, followed by a return home. The common man (plebeian), on the other hand, just received medicines!

Sound Breathing

Scientific study of meditation, which underpins many ancient health care approaches, particularly in the East, has at last rediscovered the value of slowed breathing. Four randomised controlled trials, using a biofeedback device called a RESPeRATE, [14] have shown that breathing exercises that slow the breath to about six breaths per minute, with a prolonged out-breath, significantly reduce blood pressure in those with hypertension – the reduction is equivalent in effect to two antihypertensive drugs taken regularly. Just 10 minutes of such exercises four times a week are enough to achieve this effect.

Effective Facilitation

Remarkable recoveries can occur when people re-define the relationship between themselves and the world, and create internal balance and restoration of homeostasis, where their human needs are met.

The problem for many people, however, is that in a state of struggle, both external and internal, they cannot take charge. A skilled facilitator is required to help them re-engage the observing self – the rational part of us that can see the bigger picture.

It is particularly important, therefore, that GPs use the time they have well. The standard 10-minute consultation allows a history, examination, and the consideration of tests to exclude pathology. If symptoms remain unexplained, there is a need to create more time, to help the patient see how current predicaments and challenges may have contributed to loss of homeostasis and resilience. [15]

Once such a mutual understanding is reached, this is when effective counsellors and social prescribers have a role in the GP surgery. With such help, individuals can rediscover their strengths and learn to apply appropriate choices to their lifestyle and relationships.

REFERENCES

[1] S. Wessely, C. Nimnuan, M. Sharpe, *Functional somatic syndromes: one or many?* Lancet, 1999, 354, 936–3 https://pubmed.ncbi.nlm.nih.gov/10489969/

[2] Jan van Dixhoorn, Hans Folgerin, *The Nijmegen Questionnaire and dysfunctional breathing,* ERJ Open Res. May 2015 https://openres.ersjournals.com/content/1/1/00001-2015

Rosalba Courtney, Jan van Dixhoorn, Kenneth Mark Greenwood, Els L M Anthonissen, *Medically unexplained dyspnea: partly moderated by dysfunctional (thoracic dominant) breathing pattern,* Journal of Asthma, Vol. 8, 2011 https://pubmed.ncbi.nlm.nih.gov/21341969

[3] C. Burton, *Beyond somatisation: a review of the understanding and treatment of medically unexplained physical symptoms (MUPS),* British Journal of General Practice, 2003, 53, 233–241 https://www.ncbi.nlm.nih.gov/pmc/articles/PMC1314551/

[4] T. Olde Hartman, P. Lucassen, E. van de Lisdonk, H. Bor, C. van Weel, *Chronic functional somatic symptoms: a single syndrome?* British Journal of General Practice, 2004, 54, 922–927 https://www.ncbi.nlm.nih.gov/pmc/articles/PMC1326111/

[5] K. Kroenke, R. K. Price, *Symptoms in the community. Prevalence, classification, and psychiatric co-morbidity,* Archives of Internal Medicine, 1993, 153, 2474–80 https://pubmed.ncbi.nlm.nih.gov/8215752/

[6] L-A. Martinez-Martinez, T. Mora, A. Vargas, M. Fuentes-Iniestra, M. Martínez-Lavín, *Sympathetic nervous system dysfunction in fibromyalgia, chronic fatigue syndrome, irritable bowel syndrome, and interstitial cystitis: a review of case-control studies,* Journal of Clinical Rheumatology, 2014; 20(3): 146-150 https://pubmed.ncbi.nlm.nih.gov/24662556/

[7] C. Dowrick, A. Ring, G. M. Humphris, P. Salmon, *Normalisation of unexplained symptoms by general practitioners: a functional typology,* British Journal of General Practice, 2004, 54, 165–70 https://pubmed.ncbi.nlm.nih.gov/15006120/

[8] Candice Pert, *Molecules of Emotion: Why You Feel The Way You Feel,* Simon & Schuster UK, 2012

[9] C. B. Pert, M. R. Ruff, R. J. Weber, M. Herkenham, *Neuropeptides and their receptors: a psychosomatic network,* Journal of Immunology, 1985, 135, 820–826 https://pubmed.ncbi.nlm.nih.gov/2989371/

[10] David Beales, Helen Whitten, *Emotional Healing,* Wiley, 2010

[11] A. Bullock, S. Trombley, *The New Fontana Dictionary of Modern Thought (Nixon, P, 404–405),* HarperCollins, 1999

[12] L. Chaitow, D. Bradley, C. Gilbert, *Multi-disciplinary approaches to breathing pattern disorders,* Churchill Livingstone, 2002

[13] C. Dowrick, A. Ring, G. M. Humphris, P. Salmon, *Normalisation of unexplained symptoms by general practitioners: a functional typology,* British Journal of General Practice, 2004, 54, 165–70 https://pubmed.ncbi.nlm.nih.gov/15006120/

[14] E. Grossman, A. Grossman, M. Schein, R. Zimlichman, B. Gavish, *Breathing control lowers blood pressure,* Journal of Human Hypertension, 2001, 15, 4, 263–9 https://pubmed.ncbi.nlm.nih.gov/11319675/

[15] D. Beales, *Beyond mind–body dualism: implications for patient care,* Journal of Holistic Health Care, 2004, 1, 3, 15–22

~~~~~

Supporting and Empowering Carers – Put the Feelers Out!

Sara Challice. Extract from *Who Cares? – How to care for yourself whilst caring for a loved one,* published by Hammersmith Health Books, 2020, www.hammersmithbooks.co.uk www.whocares4carers.com

~~~~~

Suddenly discovering you are a carer can be a daunting prospect. You may struggle to come to grips with the situation and the many challenges that can arise.

Many carers suffer loneliness and isolation, often because they are unable to leave their loved ones alone at home. Feelings of segregation can make us feel there is an invisible barrier between our own world and the world outside us. We might be thinking everyone else is enjoying their life whilst we have been forgotten. If we consistently have these negative thought patterns 'on a loop', this could lead to anxiety and depression. Not only this, many believe this is how life is now, and they just have to get on with it.

I believe life is what you make it, even during the most challenging times. Attempting to deal with caring solely on our own is not an option, but when it comes to looking for support, where do we turn? Sadly, there is not enough information or support for carers readily available. It took me years to discover the various channels open to support me as a carer, and support my disabled husband. The trouble is, how do you go looking for something you don't even know exists?

The trouble is, how do you go looking for something you don't even know exists?

Most of us visit local doctors or hospitals when we fall ill, but, as I discovered, even though we visited these weekly, not once were we asked if we needed help at home or if we were getting enough support. There were times when it took all my effort to get Neal all the way to hospital for a regular appointment to see his oncologist, only for the consultant to treat our appointment as a 'ticking the box' exercise. Occasionally, as I reversed Neal in his wheelchair out of the consulting room, I have even laughed and asked, 'Is that it?'

To be honest, at that time, Neal was a palliative care patient and there was little more they could do for him, but even so, offering information on support at home would have been a great help.

During Neal's final year, his oncologist suggested we could Skype his appointment, saving us the stress of coming all the way to hospital, so that's what we did. If you don't have to have blood tests and are just having a follow-up appointment, you could suggest this to your doctor, provided they have the necessary facilities.

As our doctors didn't offer advice on where we could seek support, I had to put feelers out to discover what was available in our local area. Having done so, the help we finally received was wonderful and came from various sources, but I still had to go looking for it, on top of caring full-time.

Don't suffer in silence

Many carers struggle behind closed doors. If this sounds like you, don't suffer in silence. You may have a carers' support centre nearby. I found mine invaluable. They informed me of other charities with help available to both Neal and me, also nearby. Where you live will determine what support is available to you.

There may be charities in your area that were originally founded for people with specific illnesses or conditions, but now also support those who care for them. There's no harm in calling them to find out if they can help. Even if they can't, they may know of other services in your area that could.

I have found that chatting with other carers at local charities helped me discover other services available. Other carers can provide a wealth of knowledge on what is available locally. Some years ago, a Macmillan Cancer Support specialist nurse visited Neal and me. She told us about a neurological charity down the road called Integrated Neurological Services (INS) that could support us both. Not only did INS give Neal one-to-one physiotherapy free of charge, but they supported me as his carer.

You just don't know what is available until you start looking. If you become involved with a charity, you may learn a whole lot more besides – things that could benefit both you and your loved one.

Charities and social services can give support as well as offering advice and pointing you in the direction of other available services. Check the posters and leaflets in your doctor's surgery or search online for "local charity support" and don't feel bashful about receiving charity. Many charities are contracted or receive grants from the state to help in the community, so not all money comes from donations. There may also be local or national charities specific to your needs. In addition, look for day centres nearby that could give you a regular break for a number of hours whilst your loved one is looked after.

Carers can be a fountain of knowledge on what is available in your local area

You may have heard the phrase, "If you don't ask, you don't get". Opening up and speaking to your doctor, local services, friends, family and anyone else you can think of, could help you receive more support. If a district nurse or paid carers come to your home, they will be worth asking as well. You may be pleasantly surprised to find what is available for you.

Over to you…Who can you reach out to?

• Do you have a local carers' centre and have you contacted it to see what is available for you and/or your loved one?

• Are there any other charities nearby that offer support to carers?

• Have you spoken to your doctor and healthcare specialists about what may be available to you from the state? Have you rung social services?

• If you search for charities in your local area online, are there any new charities or support groups that might be of benefit?

• Do you know of other carers you can reach out to, to discover what help and benefits they are receiving? Someone going through a similar situation to yours may have important information you would not have otherwise discovered.

~~~~~

Keeping Your Own Health Record

It is important and very useful for those with neurological conditions, the clients, to keep a copy of their health records – either on a computer or in a folder to keep letters and notes or in a purpose designed Health Record Book. This can be developed to the individual's needs and wishes. It is essential information but how it is kept is up to the individual. It gives the following benefits:

• The client is empowered by having copies of the information about them and their condition. It is a very important means of helping the client control his/her own life.

• Recording different types of intervention in chronological order and how the client responds to them, encourages him/her to take
~~~~~

responsibility, which may at times need the support of close family members or friends.

• Professionals can be shown it to understand a new client's medical history and health situation, who was involved, and the interventions already provided, so duplication could be avoided, the most effective support and treatment provided and to encourage good liaison amongst all the parties concerned.

A record of the client's level of function can be kept as a base line to monitor any improvements or deterioration, which may occur in the long-term management of neurological conditions. A further record can be kept of any problems arising and the intervention provided, also of any treatment or support meetings that have occurred with the points that the client may wish to raise regarding the outcome of a meeting.

The daily and weekly routine can be recorded so that any intervention can occur at a convenient time for the client and family member. A chart can also be kept to monitor varying symptoms and problems prevalent in some neurological conditions with the response to any intervention to see if there is any amelioration of the symptoms and problems. This can be particularly useful for people with multiple sclerosis with their varying problems and their response to medication.

Intervention can be closely monitored giving the clients response:

(1) To medication with the date, type, dose, and response, re/effectiveness, or in the case of people with Parkinson's disease this will be a way of recording and demonstrating the negative effects of the medication, e.g. hallucinations.

(2) To any type of equipment with the type, source and response, re/effectiveness or problems arising.

(3) To any therapy intervention.

This can also assist in research in all three areas, for the response of the client and their carers is of prime importance. Research in turn can also help education of how neurological conditions can be effectively supported to reach or maintain their potential for as long as possible and have an optimal quality of life for them and their carers/supporters.

An organised health record is also a useful way to pass on important information when a client needs to go into a Respite or Care Home, temporarily or permanently, or a Hospice. It covers the client's medication and at what times it needs to be taken, the equipment they may need and the exercise regime they may use to maintain range of movement and strength of muscles to allow them to perhaps move in bed as they require, encouraging some measure of independence.

A Medical Opinion

This is the assessment of a purpose designed Health Record Book given by a medical student from St George's Medical School.

The Health Record is a simple tool which has the potential for major impact. As a medical professional, many patients come to me with nothing other than a vague recollection of the key information needed to provide an adequate diagnosis and treatment plan. This is particularly complicated with certain specialties, including Neurology, in which patients may struggle from memory loss or speech difficulties.

In these cases, the Health Record Book would help to serve as a detailed account of the patient's medical history, day to day activities, and medical professionals involved in their care. Not only does this simplify the task of retrieving vital information from patients and their carers, it helps to provide a complete picture of the patient to assist us in providing them care in a holistic, patient-centred manner.

The structure of the Health Record is well organised, with distinct categories for significant information. A running diary of medical events helps put into context both the overall timeline of events and the relative time course, which is helpful in assessing the rate of a patient's progress or decline. This can help provide the impetus for key decisions in their management plan.

The inclusion of daily activities and equipment is incredibly useful information to medical professionals of all types (e.g. physiotherapists, occupational therapists, speech and language therapists, nurses, etc.), helping to maintain a regular routine and mitigate the potential for extraneous stressors. The list of medications and timetable helps in avoiding prescribing errors, assessing potential side effects, and making dosing/timing adjustments.

Though I suspect some people would struggle to maintain a complete and accurate Health Record Book, the insights that can be gained from having done so provide an invaluable tool for patients and the carers they come into contact with. My hope is that the use of this Health Record

Book becomes standard practice so that it may be distributed and used by a significant portion of the general public. This simple measure would have positive ripple effects for everyone involved.

Health Record Book – Types of Content

- People involved (names, addresses, contact numbers of family, community contacts and professionals)
- Diary of medical events (e.g. decisions made): This section should contain a concise record of events requiring hospitalisation, prolonged or acute medical intervention or otherwise of special relevance to current state of health.
- General medical history: This section should be a brief assessment by the patient of significant milestones in his/her health pathway including those in childhood. Also relevant family history (e.g. coronary disease, epilepsy, Parkinson's disease etc.)
- Allergies and immunisations
- History of present primary condition
- Diagnosis, symptoms, progression, difficulties and intervention.
- Level of function over 24 hours
- Medication/Drugs
- Medication list and timetable
- Daily activities to improve function including sleep preferences, e.g. position, pillows and eating habits
- Daily routine – Weekly routine
- Equipment date, type, source, and comments
- District nurse
- Charts (if necessary)

~~~~~

Taking Back Control Programme

Carol Williams. Carol Joined INS in 2010, in a newly created post of Senior Social Worker, with supervisory responsibility of a social worker, befriender service, supporting carers and offering placements to trainee counsellors and social workers.

~~~~~

INS developed this programme and offered it to clients and carers initially in 2011. The carers were offered an adapted version, and from this, a new Carers Support Group was established.

Since then, INS has been pleased to receive funding at intervals from the London boroughs of Hounslow and Richmond to support the operation of the programme. It is also something that INS is able to provide when other means are available, to meet the needs of clients and carers.

Aims

The aim of the programme is to work with INS clients and carers to develop coping strategies to help them regain a sense of control and perspective and to help them manage their anxiety and depression. These self-management skills help them regain and/or maintain general psychological health and enhance overall well-being. Research also indicates there is likely to be an indirect benefit to the wider network of family, friends and work colleagues.

Programme Structure

The programme comprises an eight-week closed group for clients, and a three-week closed group for carers, based on cognitive behavioural principles set out in the Mental Health Handbook by Trevor J Powell, plus individual emotional support provided by the clinical team. This programme is part of an integrated package of support offered to INS clients and carers.

The programme is led by the Senior Social Worker and Senior Occupational Therapist, supported by the social work and occupational therapy team. These clinicians are chosen because of the specialist dual training in physical and mental well-being.

An initial screening and evaluation are completed by the participants to measure the outcomes of participation and provide statistical data for analysis. The self-assessment tool used for this is the Hospital Anxiety and Depression (HAD) Scale.

Each group is a maximum of eight people.

Client Involvement

The programme was developed in response to a need expressed by clients and carers for more specialist input in addressing issues around mental well-being. These issues are recognised and well evidenced in NICE guidelines for Multiple Sclerosis, Parkinson's Disease and Stroke, as well as the NICE guidelines for Depression (Physical Disability section).

"I feel trapped inside my body . . . as if I'm not in control . . . almost as if someone or something else is running my life." (patient).

"Depression affects around 40–50% of people with PD. It is usually mild to moderate... The characteristic features of depression are low mood, loss of interest and enjoyment, and fatigue., excessive worry, feelings of worthlessness, hopelessness and guilt, negative views of self and life, and thoughts of suicide. Psychological and physical symptoms of anxiety are also common. The development of depression creates an added burden for people with PD and their carers and has been shown to be an important determinant of quality of life" [1]

The programme is able to address individual needs and issues, working towards enabling each participant to develop the strategies needed to self-manage their symptoms of anxiety, stress and depression to enhance their overall well-being. Through sharing the experience in a small group setting, participants are able to learn from and support each other.

Each session provides a focus on different symptoms and emotions, and the possible strategies that could be implemented to work towards self-management. Specific tasks are set each week for completion between group sessions to enhance the learning of self-awareness and self-management. Copies of the materials used are provided to the participants for their use during the programme and for their ongoing self-management.

Following completion of the programme, each participant is offered individual follow-up support on a 1:1 basis and referred to other services for more specific support, as appropriate.

Outcomes For Individuals

- Increased sense of coping and being in control of their situation
- Improved mood with fewer feelings of anxiety or depression
- Increased knowledge in self-management, using a range of skills and strategies to cope
- Increased sense of self-awareness and control
- Increased confidence, self-esteem and overall well-being

• Improved quality of life through maintaining independence, social involvement and family relationships
• Increased sense of being supported

Potential Long-Term Wider Benefits

• Improved adjustment to their condition, reducing the burden on the carer, reliance on services, use of medication and unnecessary hospital admission
• Sustaining independence and social participation
• Minimise further deterioration in mental health
• Possible reduction in emergency care support resulting from inability of carer to continue with caring role
• Improved quality of life for family, friends and work colleagues.

[1] Quotes from NICE PD guidance

~~~~~

Mind, Body, and Spirit Group

Sara Challice

~~~~~

When looking to improve health, we not only need to focus on the physical body, but also on the mind and the spirit. Within this INS group, we look at many ways to empower yourself and to boost mental and physical health.

The group is diverse, with a number of different nationalities and faiths – but we all come together to explore ways to improve health and learn more on the meaning and purpose of life.

The session starts with EFT (Emotional Freedom Technique), tapping on the meridian lines in the body to restore balance to the body's energy. We feel into the energy of our body, noticing how we feel before and after this technique. We then close our eyes and meditate together, as we go through a "body scan", relaxing the body and noticing where we may feel tense so as to breathe in and relax further.

At the beginning of the session, we take the names of anyone that we would like to send love and healing light to. This also includes anyone in the group would also like to be added. These names are then read out at the end of the meditation, as we all send love and healing to those who need it.

Many elements and topics discussed, include:

- Health
- Holistic approaches to improve wellbeing
- Relaxation
- Nutrition
- Exercise
- Video clips
- Books
- Philosophy
- Poetry
- Science
- Research
- Religion
- Personal experiences

As well as discussing and sharing the above, we look to see how we can bring more joy into our day, raising our frequency, and living more in the present and in love – rather than in fear.

The group is also supportive and all-encompassing. Whenever someone is struggling with certain issues, whether it be physical health or dynamics in the family, or something else, we look to help support and offer advice.

Because many in the group have already researched into health and well-being, looking to see what is available to us, many bring information from doctors, scientists and authors, including:

- Eckhart Tolle, with his book *The Power of Now*. Eckhart was depressed for many years, but then one night, had an epiphany, changing him forever. A German-born spiritual teacher and self-help author, he gives many talks to help us live in the present and help relieve suffering. "Observe your thoughts. Don't believe in them." www.eckharttolle.com

- Anita Moorjani, with her book, *Dying To Be Me*. Author and speaker, Anita had an NDE, Near Death Experience, whilst living with end stage cancer. She came back and healed in weeks, which was all documented. "Love yourself like your life depends on it, because it does." www.anitamoorjani.com

• Dr Joe Dispenza, with his book *You are the Placebo.* After becoming badly injured in a cycle race, Joe chose to use meditation and visualisation to heal himself. In overcoming his injuries, he chose to spend the rest of his life researching the mind body connection.

"Life is about management of energy. Where you place your attention is where you place your energy." www.drjoedispenza.com

• Dr Bruce Lipton, with his book *The Biology of Belief.* An American developmental biologist noted for his views on epigenetics. He claims that beliefs control human biology rather than DNA and inheritance. "The moment you change your perception is the moment you rewrite the chemistry of your body." www.brucelipton.com

• Wayne Dyer, with his book *Change Your Thoughts, Change Your Life.* An American self-help author and a motivational speaker. "You cannot always control what goes on outside, but you can always control what goes on inside." www.drwaynedyer.com

• Gary Zukav, with his book *Seat of the Soul.* American spiritual teacher. Has appeared more than 30 times on The Oprah Winfrey Show to discuss transformation in human consciousness concepts. "Eventually, you will come to understand that love heals everything, and love is all there is." www.seatofthesoul.com

• Dr Eben Alexander, with his book *Proof of Heaven.* American neurosurgeon and author. Had a near-death experience in 2008, under medically-induced coma when treated for meningitis, experiencing the afterlife. "Laughter and irony are at heart reminders that we are not prisoners in this world, but voyagers through it." www.ebenalexander.com

• Gregg Braden, with his book *The Divine Matrix.* American New Age author, linking science and spirituality. "There can only be one solution to any problem: a change in attitude and in consciousness." www.greggbraden.com

After each session, the group receive a synopsis of all books, links and information discussed during the session, allowing for further reading and insights if they want to know more to help benefit their own health and well-being.

At the time of going to print, the Mind, Body, and Spirit group includes the INS founder, published authors, a retired GP, teachers, a Mindfulness instructor and reiki masters.

~~~~~
~~~~~

Chapter 9
Fruits of Experience – Important Messages

1. Early Diagnosis and Assessment

It is important to have a diagnosis and assessment as early as possible. Early warning signs are often missed but knowledge of early signs and symptoms will support the person to understand what is going on and make informed choices about their lifestyle.

Caught early the person can be taught to counteract the effect of the disease before the abnormalities become a habit which are harder to change.

Stroke

• face – weakness on one side
• weakness on one side of the body affecting arm and leg – which may affect sensation
• speech – may be slurred
• sudden loss or blurring of vision
• difficulty understanding
• confusion
• severe headache
• loss of balance
• loss of coordination
• dizziness

Parkinson's

• disturbances of sleep rhythms
• sluggish bowels
• bent posture
• lack of arm swing on one side
• mask like facial features, due to stiffness in the facial muscles, which can lead to the assumption from others that the person is not engaging with conversations
• general slowness without the characteristic tremor.

Multiple Sclerosis

- numbness, tingling, alteration in skin sensation
- reduced muscle power, muscle stiffness and spasms
- problems with balance and coordination
- fatigue
- difficulty walking
- vision problems, blurred vision, double vision
- sexual problems
- bowel and bladder problems
- problems with thinking, learning and planning.
- slurred speech

Call an ambulance if there are signals of sudden loss of control of a body part or sudden loss of speech or other signals of nervous system damage. A reduced response time from onset of symptoms may lead to delay in receiving clot busting drugs and reduced damage to the brain.

The day of diagnosis is hugely important for someone with a neurological condition and for their family. [See p74 and p174 for the response of doctors as patients] A family member should be present when the diagnosis is given. Here is where the neurologist must help the person to be proactive in coping with the condition so that it does not dictate their lifestyle. The person needs to be supported mind, body and spirit, the latter being the most important otherwise the person can go into a depression and have a detrimental effect on the family. They need to understand their diagnosis, they need to learn how to counteract the effects of the disease physically and they need to learn strategies to help them cope with a diagnosis which will vary as is also necessary for their family.

After the diagnosis has been given, the person may "need to grieve for the person they were" so they can come to terms with what is happening to them.

Once the diagnosis has been accepted, the person then needs to be supported to see how they can deal positively with the situation, and be prepared to move on with their life.

Michael J. Fox is a wonderful example of rising to the challenge of a diagnosis of Parkinson's early in his career as an actor to be able to continue and then raise millions of dollars for research into this condition.

His guiding principle is "Live in the moment, enjoy the day make the most of what you have". [1]

2. Immediate and Ongoing Responses to the Presenting Difficulties

The presenting difficulties need to be immediately addressed by

- An explanation of the condition
- Emotional strategies to give the person hope and encouragement.
- Strategies such as education to teach the person how to help themselves

Similar to an athlete in continuous training for their sport, someone with a disability must prepare their mind, body, and spirit for their day so that they can really enjoy it and carry out what they need and wish to do. Their race is for a good quality of life for them and their family.

Early Intervention

Depending on the damage, an early intervention should be started where the patient is, (e.g. in the bed) to help them move more independently to make themselves comfortable through therapy which encompasses movement, speech and function helping them to understand what has happened and how they can help themselves.

If the nurses can be guided to move the limbs and the body in as normal a way as possible by giving instructions to the patient in the first person singular (some patients in a coma can still hear the spoken word [2]), with repetition the patient may start to respond actively. An important aim is to maintain a normal range of movement to prevent contractures.

Supporting and Maintaining Functionality

It is important to:

- have good balance in standing and sitting
- maintain as full range of movement as possible
- strengthen core control

To do this the person will need to relearn how to function optimally.

- Gentle stretching and moving before getting out of bed will warm the muscles and help to prepare the person for the day. [See Appendix 1 – Basic Morning Programme to Prepare for the Day]

• If facial muscles are affected, it is very important to stretch the muscles and maintain facial expression for better social interaction, with the ability to smile.

• Getting out of a chair or bed can become difficult, so it is important to teach the person how to use their body well, ensuring that the head comes forward over their toes when standing up and sitting down. When sitting and relaxing, it is important that the person learns to put their weight onto the affected side to stimulate the muscles over the shoulder, whilst at times, stretching their fingers or clasping their hands together which helps stretch the fingers. [See Appendix 2, Photo 1, clasped hands]

• When getting ready to stand up, prepare for this by expanding the diaphragm as you breath in and move as you breath out.

• A good strategy is to create a rhythm to the day – giving time for preparation, work and rest. Also, not only is one nurtured with appropriate food, but also with mental stimulation.

A Good Diet

Dr Craig Hassed, in his book *The Essence of Health: the Seven Pillars of Wellbeing,* highlights how important this is; *"Food as medicine has a vital part to play in health maintenance and management".* [3] [The Pillars are: Education; Stress Management; Spirituality; Exercise; Nutrition; Connectedness; Environment]

By eating vegetables and fruit containing minerals, vitamins and fibre with proteins such as lean meat, fish, eggs, peas, beans, lentils with nuts and seeds which contain chemicals to regulate thoughts and feelings, this can help mental and physical health plus provide more energy and help reduce depression. Keeping well hydrated reduces constipation. For people with Parkinson's if taking L-Dopa, it is important to take the medication 30 minutes before eating as protein reduces the effective absorption of this important drug.

Emotional Well-Being

Emotional well-being can be overlooked but is critical to enable the person to be as well as they can be. Teaching videos can be found in many places including on the web and in the form of apps. YouTube teachings and resources by Thich Nhat Hanh and other teachers such as Eckhart Tole provide guidance. *"The gift of learning to meditate is the greatest gift you can give yourself"*. [4]

Regular time for mindfulness or meditation and an awareness of the importance of living in the present moment are very helpful. When Michael J. Fox was in Bhutan, a country which was the birthplace of "Gross National Happiness" where the main religion is Buddhism focussing on compassion, contentment and calmness, he noticed that his Parkinsonian symptoms had markedly reduced. [5]

INS' Mind, Body, and Spirit group is all-encompassing and holistic, helping those with neurological conditions and carers, of all faiths and backgrounds. The group supports them mentally, emotionally, physically and spiritually. Even when living with a life-long health condition, there is always more we can do to empower ourselves so as to improve the quality of life, health and wellbeing.

Because many in the group have already researched into health and well-being, we share information that is readily available from doctors, scientists and authors, sharing books, videos and upcoming talks. We recognise that there is more than just the physical world, connecting to a greater power, and focusing on the present moment, which helps to relieve suffering, bringing about more peace and joy.

Guidance and Information

The person and their family will need a social work assessment and support as they learn how to negotiate the social care system, especially in complex situations. Where the situation is complex, they will need ongoing care and support to find the best help in a timely fashion. This intervention needs to have ongoing monitoring with Health and Social Services to ensure that the service is beneficial for the person and their family as well as cost effective.

Information can be found from relevant support organisations, e.g. the Stroke Association, Parkinson's UK, the Multiple Sclerosis Society, the Motor Neurone Disease Association, etc. [See Sources of Information, p207] [See also Appendix 4 – Advice for People with Neurological Conditions]

3. Importance of a Personal Health Record

As a person's health changes it can be difficult to remember what has happened – what were the problems, who were the professionals involved, and what was the response, e.g. some medication can cause hallucinations and an increased likelihood to addiction such as gambling. The person should be encouraged to keep their own record. They can record:

- who is involved in their medical care with dates
- their past medical history
- their presenting medical condition
- the medication they take with their response to it
- any therapy that is given and progress if any
- equipment provided and by whom
- daily routine
- diet changes and impact
- exercise, routines, and impact
- care and support and how provided
- drug history
- record of the medication to take and the timing in relation to food intake which is especially important for people with Parkinson's

This should help ensure that the person's medication and physical needs are understood if they need to be admitted to hospital, respite or hospice care. One of the aims of this medical file is that it may help the rehabilitation service find the most efficient and effective way to support such people and their family from diagnosis onwards as it lends itself to audit analysis. [6]

A holistic medical assessment based on the Lawrence Weed format with the acronym SOAP as a guide – S = Subjective history; O = Objective findings; A = Analysis; P = Plan – and a description of a typical day describing the positive actions that lead to a sense of improved well-being is helpful. Then identify ongoing problems and list them with room to describe the approaches that have helped or hindered progress. [7]

4. The Value of Working in Groups

Meeting other people in a caring environment can be very supportive. Working with people with the same diagnosis can foster a feeling of solidarity enabling people to share issues and challenges. Together people can often find solutions by sharing how they cope. Together they have a vested interested in finding ways to resolve issues.

• Self-help therapy groups where an initial social session leads to therapy to help prepare them for the day to cope in the different situation met throughout a day – in sitting, lying, standing and walking with ways of learning to improve the tasks they are finding difficult to do, e.g. writing.

• The therapy sessions can then lead to different activities which can help in confidence building, finding new avenues of interest, e.g. creative writing, yoga, art, music etc. This will also help people feel less isolated in an environment where there is guidance and support.

• One-to-one sessions can be run to improve the individual's response in the group session, which is a preparation for the day either at home or at work. For example, speech; either individual coaching or a speech-aphasic group, or a play reading group to improve confidence and vocal production.

5. Get Out and About in your Local Community

People should be encouraged and supported to get out into their local communities to continue to enjoy activities that they loved, to try something new on their own, or in organised outings.

Outings can also be arranged to different environments such as going to the theatre, going to a park, going to shops. Relatives are encouraged to join the participants so they, the therapy staff, and volunteers can learn how to support the person in the community.

Individual participants can be supported to relearn activities such as using buses and trains which often entail using an escalator. Once they are confident then this can lead to greater independence and possibly return to work or finding another more suitable occupation. A great example of this is "Jackie" who came to INS unable to use public transport. An occupational therapist took Jackie into the community and taught her how to cope with the underground, which involved escalators. Jackie was then independently able to visit her family, who lived on the other side of London, a few years after her stroke.

When people with neurological conditions get out into their local community it not only helps them in not feeling isolated but also gives the community itself a greater understanding of disability, and how disabled people can be assimilated, accepted, and valued; e.g. the Paralympic Games and the Invictus Games.

6. Groups for Carers

Family and friends provide the most support for most people with disabilities, and, as carers, their health and well-being is of paramount importance. Carer groups are extremely helpful, providing necessary support in a safe environment for the family member. This helps them feel open to discuss anything with people who understand their present circumstances. Here, their well-being is nurtured with opportunities for mutual learning in how to support the whole family in a holistic way. Sara Challice's book *Who Cares?* recounts her experience as a carer and is a valuable guide to avoiding stress and burnout. [8]

7. Crucial Needs

• For a Neurological team both in Hospital and in the Community to liaise closely with Social Services. This will create a way of understanding the whole journey of people with neurological conditions from diagnosis onwards to help them and the family member have as a good a quality of life as possible. The team will also utilise the skills of the different members of the team – neurologists, GPs, nurses, physiotherapists, occupational therapists, speech and language therapists, dieticians, psychologists, bioengineers, technicians, physiologists, counsellors, carers, managers – where there is sometimes the need to address complex problems.

This will help the person reach and maintain potential for as long as possible thus reducing the cost of unnecessarily increasing dependence and mental health problems. It will be a way of monitoring their journey to find the most effective and efficient way of supporting them. This will help to provide best practice to standardise care and support across the country. There is a need to liaise with hospitals, care homes, and hospices, to plan ahead to avoid unnecessary problems, e.g. contractures and emergency admissions. It is very valuable to have respite availability to give the family carer a break. Their health record should be explained to the staff to ensure the person's regime is maintained to avoid deterioration.

• Health and Social Services together determine a personal budget based on the person's care and support needs. This budget can either commission support or be given to the person to manage themselves. The benefits of the person managing themselves is that they can recruit and employ carers. The carers can be trained specifically for the person they are supporting. Initially Social Services provides the funding but as the condition progresses Health funding can become available to help them reach and maintain their potential for as long as possible, to help them have optimal independence and prevent unnecessary disability. This can also be managed by the person which allows for support to continue to be provided by carers who the person knows.

• People with long-term neurological conditions – this should include people with mental illness, cerebral palsy and learning difficulties – may need ongoing support for life. Here it is very important to achieve a fulfilling life despite the condition. A good example is given by Professor Jelinek who himself has MS and has written Overcoming MS from personal experience. [3] Coping strategies may need to be organised in advance with ongoing monitoring to find the most effective and efficient way of supporting such people and their families. This includes their opinion and ideas to enhance harmony in living and dying.

8. An Education Resource

Developing a learning environment within a community neuro team can provide a wide variety of students working and learning together – physiotherapists, occupational therapists, speech and language therapists, social work students, and medical students – with the opportunity to listen to the experiences of patients, their families, and their carers, and give them an understanding of the two sides of the same situation. This can give students the opportunity to visit people with neuro conditions in their own surroundings which may stimulate an interest in research to prove the value of different therapies.

9. Research and Audit

Where research is undertaken with patients the aims should be discussed with them to ensure that their involvement and cooperation has been considered. Research questions should be instrumental in directing the way forward considering previous research findings so that positive findings are brought into present practice. The knowledge gained from the money, time, and people's involvement is used to direct the way forward in the future.

Collaboration needs to be made and maintained with the different societies for people with neurological conditions such as, the Stroke Association, Parkinson's UK, the Multiple Sclerosis Society, the Motor Neurone Disease Association, etc. to learn about and pass on relevant information. [See Sources of Information]

~~~~~

May all be happy.
May all be without disease.
May all creatures have well-being.
And none be in misery of any sort.
Peace, peace, peace

An ancient invocation as spoken by Nelson Mandela at his inauguration as President of South Africa.

REFERENCES

[1] Michael J. Fox, the *Back to the Future* star who was diagnosed with Parkinson's in 1991, has published his fourth book: *No Time Like the Future: An Optimist Considers Mortality*, Headline Publishing Group, 2020

[2] Anita Moorjani, *Dying To Be Me*, Hay House UK, 2012

[3] Dr Craig Hassed, *The Essence of Health: the Seven Pillars of Wellbeing*, Ebury Australia, 2008

Professor George Jelinek, *Overcoming Multiple Sclerosis*, Allen & Unwin, 2016 https://overcomingms.org/about-us/professor-george-jelinek

[4] *The Best of Thich Nhat Hanh: Life, Teachings, Quotes, and Books*, Lion's Roar Foundation, 2021 https://www.lionsroar.com/thich-nhat-hanh/

[5] *Fox found solace in Bhutan*, Daily Star, 1 April 2009 https://www.dailystar.co.uk/showbiz/fox-found-solace-in-bhutan-18063506

[6] *Interview with Lawrence Weed, MD* – The Father of the Problem-Oriented Medical Record Looks Ahead, The Permanente Journal, Vol. 13, No. 3, 2009 https://www.ncbi.nlm.nih.gov/pmc/articles/PMC2911807/
~~~~~

[7] *Lawrence Leonard Weed,* The Lancet, Vol. 390, Issue 10093, p450, July 29, 2017 https://www.thelancet.com/journals/lancet/article/PIIS0140-6736(17)31911-6/fulltext

[8] Sara Challice, *Who Cares? – How to care for yourself whilst caring for a loved one,* Hammersmith Health Books, 2020

~~~~~
~~~~~

PART 4

THE CREATION OF A CHARITY

Integrated Neurological Services (INS)
https://www.ins.org.uk/

Chapter 10
Why & How INS was Formed

Eleanor Kinnear

"You can give a hungry man a fish to eat, but if you teach him how to fish he will have food for life"

WHY.....

The Need for Rehabilitation

Eleanor (Ellie) Kinnear is a chartered physiotherapist with neurological experience through clinical practice and research. [1] Early in her career several incidents dramatically drew her attention to the importance of certain aspects of rehabilitation.

In 1963, when she was working in Switzerland at the clinic in Bad Ragaz, one of her patients in her mid-twenties, who had had an aneurism resulting in a stroke, was told by her doctor that the condition she was now in would not improve. Since patients are not monitored once out of hospital, how can a doctor give such a prognosis? After being told this, the patient had a nervous breakdown. [2]

Another patient in this clinic, was a young man, who had sustained a head injury while steeple-chasing, resulting in a hemiplegia, a stroke. His fiancée's family had told the fiancée that she should not marry a cripple, and the marriage was called off. Thus he lost vital support at this very vulnerable time. He actually made a good physical recovery, but was traumatised for life and went off to the wilds of Australia.

While still in Switzerland, working at the Orthopaedic Hospital of St Gallen, Ellie had a patient, who at the age of twenty-one, pregnant with her second child, had suffered a stroke. It was apparent that such a patient needed ongoing therapy, with emphasis on self-help in order for her to reach her maximum potential. Support needed to be given also to her husband and recent father at this vulnerable time.

From these cases arose awareness of (a) the need for rehabilitation so that patients reach their potential and maintain it for as long as possible, (b) the need to educate doctors and address the power of the psychology of positive interaction with a patient whose diagnosis anyone including a doctor might experience, and (c) the importance of supporting the family members at the time of diagnosis.

Introduction to the Conductive Approach to Rehabilitation

In the early 1970s Ellie worked as a physiotherapist on an acute medical ward at Queen Mary's Hospital, Roehampton. Queen Mary's had a reputation for rehabilitation. It had a 40-bedded ward to rehabilitate people with a wide variety of disabilities with a multi-disciplinary team and was able to attract funding for innovative practices and research.

Ellie attended a lecture on Conductive Education for a child with athetoid cerebral palsy given by Ester Cotton, [3] a Danish physiotherapist. Ester had discovered this new approach for patients with neurological conditions when she visited the Peto Institute for Conductive Education in Budapest, Hungary, while working at the Bobath Centre for children with cerebral palsy.

Conductive Education is based on the principle of neuroplasticity, the process by which the brain creates new pathways for sending messages to the body, rerouting around damaged paths. New pathways are created when individuals are taught how to perform everyday tasks such as walking by breaking the task down into more achievable parts, like weightbearing and bending alternating legs.

At the lecture Ester showed a child with cerebral athetosis who was sitting on a ladder chair with his hands gripping the rung of another ladder chair at shoulder height which had been placed in front of him. He was asked to repeat "I see two hands" and then the hands stayed in place as he was asked to count to five. Maybe for the first time he was seeing and being aware of his own hands. Normally, he had no feeling for or control over his hands; his arms would be folded upwards with the hands at shoulder level. Thus, he was starting to learn hand-eye control. [For illustration of a ladder chair see Appendix 3 – Use of a Ladder Chair]

After the lecture Ellie went up to Ester to ask if this method using movement and speech might be useful for people with a stroke and speech problems. Ester said it would be applicable for such stroke patients and that she could visit Queen Mary's Hospital once a month, since with great good fortune the hospital was on her regular way to Ingfield Manor, a residential centre for children with cerebral palsy using this Conductive Education approach.

Later, Ester explained that when she had visited the Peto Institute in Budapest she saw a group of children walk down the corridor counting aloud, utterly concentrating on walking the way they had been taught. Ester looked for the conductor but no one was there. This demonstrated that the children were inspired to continue unsupervised what they had learnt.

Stroke Group Set-up at Queen Mary's Hospital, Roehampton

In 1977 Ester came regularly once a month to Queen Mary's to assist in developing a Conductive Education programme for a small group of people with a stroke. While doing this she suggested it would be good to run a whole day for the group to work on preparing for the rhythm of the day. The rehabilitation gym was available and the Friends of Queen Mary's Hospital provided a cold lunch for the patients and the supporting team which included physios, an occupational therapist, a speech and language therapist, a remedial assistant, and nurses.

The programme included an initial social time when patients arrived from the wards and from the community, then work included a programme for mobility and perceptual tasks sitting at a table tennis table, the programme continued in free sitting, standing, walking, and lying. Those patients who could help, assisted in preparing the table for lunch, all joining in to eat, when the patients could be observed socialising and how they were able to use the cutlery.

After lunch the patients could have a rest then they were assisted as necessary to go onto the floor to do a programme emphasising good posture, mobilising all limbs with the unaffected hand clasping the weaker hand and ending in being taught how to get up from the floor, standing up to then go to sit at a table for very welcome refreshments.

Ester led the programme as she had been taught at the Institute and the therapists and nurses assisted as required. Patients were taught how to prepare for movement using language and rhythm to aid memory. They were also being taught how to relax in normal positions of relaxation, which emphasised good weightbearing and stretching of muscles and joints.

Above all they were learning to function in a positive welcoming atmosphere which was conducive to learning. Physical progress was seen and also in the area of communication, comprehension and confidence. The patients found it very encouraging to see each other improve. Some people with multiple sclerosis (MS) were also included in the group.

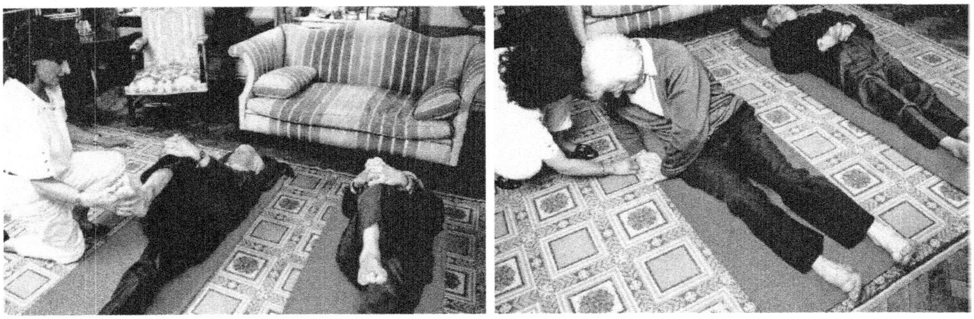

Early Stroke Group: Mobilising Lower Limbs and Weightbearing on Affected Arm

One of the people with MS invited Ellie to dinner and during the evening she told her guests how she had difficulty in getting off the toilet. Then she related how she suddenly remembered what she had been taught in the group where she had learnt to repeat the series of instructions for performing this task "I bring my feet back, I lean forwards, and I stand up", thus demonstrating how useful she found using speech and repetition in the sessions.

Importance of Groups

This Conductive approach focuses on self-help, well-being and confidence building in all aspects of rehabilitation. The main work is carried out in groups.

A group is led by a new kind of professional – a conductor – who uses a programme involving speech, movement and function together for both children and adults. Typically, the programme has a theme such as "Preparing for the Day" which would include sessions in sitting, lying, standing, and walking with functional activities and a social time at the beginning and end of the programme.

The support varies according to the individual's ability and actions taught to patients are kept as simple as possible so they more easily learn how to carry out the task independently, learning how to help themselves.

The value of the groups lies in the opportunity of the members to meet and support others in similar circumstances; to learn from each other's difficulties and successes, to share information and to develop mutual trust and make new friends; thus they are able to do things outside the group: e.g. go on holidays and outings such as companion cycling where a bicycle is shared [See photo p169]. Thus their family members and supporters can also find new friends and mutual support.

Obtaining Conductive Expertise

The main centre for training in Conductive Education is the Peto Institute for Conductive Education in Budapest. In Britain conductors are trained at NICE (National Institute of Conductive Education) in Birmingham.

A physiotherapy journal published in Hong Kong dedicated a whole edition to the value of the Conductive Education to indicate the significance of this approach for the neurologically impaired and disabled. [4] Anita Tatlow, the editor, said that *"the approach is built around the person's personality and by respecting the person's dignity and right to be active, the person will become motivated and will feel responsible for himself and his movements"*.

Vital Role of Repetition

For a skill to be learnt, the action desired needs to be practised accurately and repeated many times throughout the day before it can be carried out automatically. [5] In order for this to be achieved whoever is supporting the disabled person needs to be aware of the correct action to ensure that it is carried out in the optimum way.

Thus everyone in the rehabilitation team, physiotherapist, occupational therapist, speech and language therapist, nurse, family and social worker needs to assist in reinforcing the correct action.

Research Related Experience

An Assessment Tool

In the 1970s Ellie joined a Neuromotor group. Here was a wonderful gathering of people in professions all involved with the condition of a stroke; neurologists, speech and language therapists, occupational therapists, physiotherapists, bioengineers, technicians, psychologists and physiologists. From this gathering of over 40 professionals, an assessment tool was created, A Physical Assessment for Stroke Patients, [6] providing objective inter-related, reliably-tested measurements. This was used in the battery of assessments for patients in the pedobarograph trial. [See below]

Another important result of the Neuromotor group was produced by Marian Huett, a physiologist, She wrote the rationale for using the lying programme from a physiological point of view. [See Appendix 1 – Basic Morning Programme to Prepare for the Day] She also wrote out the physiological rationale for the use of the ladder chair in retraining walking, which involves the use of both arms. [See Appendix 3 – Use of a Ladder Chair]

Research 1 – The Controlled Trial of Physiotherapy and Occupational Therapy for Parkinson's

In 1979 Dr Brian Gibberd, one of the neurologists at Queen Mary's Hospital, asked Ellie to be involved in the first controlled trial to be set up to investigate the use of physiotherapy and occupational therapy for out-patients with Parkinson's. The patients attended for one-on-one treatment sessions eight times in four weeks.

The outcome was that the patients did not seem to improve with out-patient intervention, but therapy might help those with rapidly deteriorating conditions.

Several questions arose: was the therapy relevant or not? was the frequency of treatment sufficient or not? was the treatment given in the right environment or not? what was the opinion of the patients and their family, the most important people?

The findings were published in the British Medical Journal. [7]

Research 2 – Three-Year Trial – Retraining Standing Balance in Recent Stroke Patients by the Use of a Pedobarograph

Ellie was involved as physiotherapist in this three-year trial (1979-1982) to investigate the use of a pedobarograph, a type of biofeedback apparatus, to retrain standing balance for people in the first three months post stroke. [8] A pedobarograph is a device that records pressures exerted by the foot on contact with the ground. It measures the pressure distribution on the base of the foot. [See diagram] The trial was conducted at the Bioengineering Centre, University College, London, within the grounds of Queen Mary's Hospital, Roehampton.

Each patient was assessed with a battery of tests with a numerical score covering motor, sensory, perceptual and mental function to see how each person had responded in relation to the effect of the stroke. This holistic battery of tests gave a truly rounded understanding of where the abnormalities lay and so treatment could be directed more precisely to deal with them; e.g. one patient did not have the correct awareness of the vertical in sitting or standing, thus treatment could be directed to correcting such a basic problem for the patient.

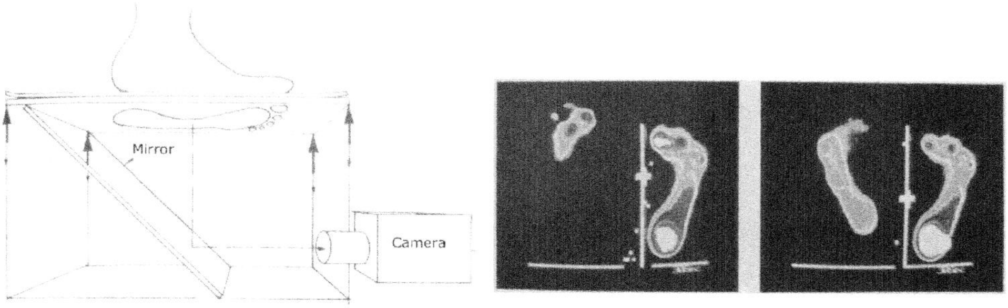

Pedobarogram and Images: Left before treatment. Right after treatment

Two patients had very similar results from the battery of tests – one was put into the experimental group and the other into the control group. The one in the experimental group made a remarkable recovery in regaining some control of his knee and the ability to lift up his toes. [See Pedobarogram images before and after treatment]

The treatment involved the use of a splint [See photo] created by a bioengineer to allow normal flexion and extension with a device to fix the knee in extension, this allowed the patient to concentrate on keeping control around his hip while working on a variety of tasks.

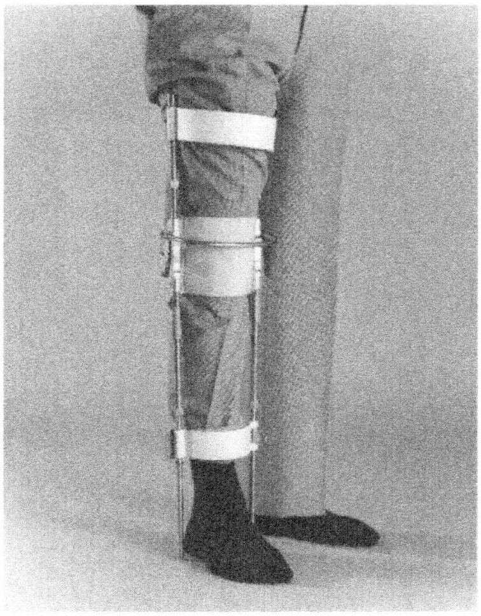

Before the end of the ten sessions (each session lasted for a maximum of 30 minutes) the patient recovered enough control around his knee to dispense with the splint. He was able to practise all the tasks in the last two days. In addition the weightbearing on his affected, weaker limb, especially on the heel of the foot stretched the muscles around the foot allowing the weaker muscles to be stimulated and he regained some control over the movement of his toes which helps in walking. The patient in the control group made little progress in the return of muscle power.

The report was shown to Professor John Basmajian at McMasters University, Ontario, Canada. He was the world expert on biofeedback. He sent her a letter stating that this could be a very important part of rehabilitation for the patient with a stroke. Here is a quote from the letter.

> *Dear Ms. Kinnear:*
> *.... I am most impressed by the intelligence and thoroughness of the study and the clarity and balance of the report. Your conclusions are careful and the cautious hope you express is warranted. Indeed, the technique has considerable potential and further larger studies of therapeutic use are justifiable even as the pedobarograph finds wider usage as an assessment tool in rehabilitation settings.*
> John V. Basmajian, M.D. Professor of Medicine, Director, Rehabilitation Centre

Six copies of the report were sent to the Department of Health. However there was no response from the people who had provided the money, nor was there any formal discussion of how the knowledge gained could be used in the clinical field.

A Good Result

After the trial in 1982 she returned to work on a medical ward at Queen Mary's Hospital when she had the opportunity to work with someone with a recent stroke, whose arm was affected, having no elbow, wrist extension or finger movement.

Using her experience of prolonged weightbearing on the affected leg in the pedobarograph trial producing stimulation of the anti-gravity muscles and inhibition of the plantar flexors, Ellie taught the patient to weightbear on the elbow when sitting, and with the elbow and wrist extended and fingers outstretched on a table when standing.

She also asked the nursing staff and the relatives of the patient to encourage him to weightbear in a normal manner as much as possible. Ten days after his stroke, the house doctor asked how was the patient improving. In fact, that day the patient was showing some elbow and wrist extension. This confirmed her belief of the importance of weightbearing with stretching joints around the wrist and ankle when patients should be encouraged to take up positions of relaxation as "normally" as possible, actions which are automatic for non-affected people. [See Appendix 2 – Normal Positions to Support Muscles & Joints for illustrations of good weightbearing and how it can be practised]

Involvement with Parkinson's

In 1986 Ellie was involved through the Parkinson's Disease Society (now known as Parkinson's UK) in a group collaboration with different professional disciplines to look at Parkinson's from a therapeutic perspective.

As a result of this collaboration two physiotherapy journals published editions wholly centred on articles about Parkinson's disease written by those involved. They included an article written by Ellie under the title Long-term management of Parkinson's disease and an article about the physiology of Parkinson's disease by Dr Marian Huett. [9]

A Working Holiday Treating People with Parkinson's

In 1987 Ellie was asked by Mary Baker, chief executive of the Parkinson's Disease Society, to provide physiotherapy for 15 patients funded by the Society to go on a two-week holiday to a specially adapted holiday home at Crab Hill run by the Society. This was the patients' first opportunity to have any physiotherapy.

Since there were 15 patients, it was decided that another physiotherapist, Elizabeth (Liz) Anderton, experienced in neurology, would help Ellie treat them in a group. Ellie had experience of working with stroke patients in a group using the Conductive Education approach. All this gave the opportunity to be with the patients over the 24 hours, providing great insight into the effect of the prescribed drugs, which may cause fluctuations during the day and the importance of taking the medication at the right time. Some of the guests responded well to having a lumbar support when eating and when travelling in a bus to various outings.

The patients seemed to respond to this approach. One guest objected to being asked to repeat what the task was before executing the action. He said it was demeaning and that he was being talked down to. It was explained to him this was done so another part of the brain might help improve his ability to function e.g. fine hand control. He then agreed to continue with the programme.

The holiday also gave the therapists a chance to try hydrotherapy with some of the guests using the Bad Ragaz Ring Method. The guests responded well to hydrotherapy which is an aquatic version of Proprioceptive Neuromuscular Facilitation (PNF). PNF had been developed from the work of Dr Kabat and the physiotherapist Maggie

Knott, who had looked very closely at how muscles work. They found out that muscles work involving a combination of abduction or adduction, flexion or extension, internal or external rotation. Thus the muscles were rehabilitated in the way that nature intended.

Realising she needed to know more about leading a group for people with Parkinson's Ellie visited the National Institute of Conductive Education in Birmingham, where she watched a Parkinson's group run by an experienced Peto-trained conductor. She was amazed by the holistic programme, where rhythm and counting were such an important part of the group session, which included a lying programme, a sitting programme, standing and walking with speech and writing – all in the space of an hour and a half. Thus different parts of the body and brain were used, all aiming at improving the activities of daily living through increasing self-confidence and self-esteem.

Community Physiotherapist

Ellie moved into a job as a community physiotherapist, where she now had the opportunity to see the reality of the lives of people with neuro conditions and its effect on their family in their home setting. They seemed to be waiting for the support team to arrive with the rest of the day in limbo. A fifth of her time was spent as the first community physiotherapist at Queen Mary's Hospital to work officially with people with learning difficulties, both in their homes and in Normansfield, a residential hospital for people with learning difficulties.

Here she was amazed at how many Normansfield residents had conditions with neurological problems, and she was also struck by how many were sitting and lying immobile in very abnormal postures for long periods. This prompted her and a physiotherapy colleague, Linda Eve, to write a paper in the Physiotherapy Journal, *Does the Wheelchair Fit?* [10] They came to the conclusion that the wheelchairs did not support the 23 patients adequately and due to the length of time that each person stayed in their chair, varying from two to 15 hours with a mean of seven hours, 20 patients had contractures leading to varying degrees of asymmetry (abnormal positions).

With her experience of Conductive Education, Ellie started a weekly group in Normansfield Hospital with permission of Val Macey, the head occupational therapist, who became involved in the group.

Ellie gradually learnt that some of the members were intelligent and articulate. At the end of a session one of the participants when asked what he felt about the session, said "It was time well spent". Another patient, who had epilepsy, spent most of the time sitting slumped in a chair, heavily drugged. While helping him to walk in a more normal way, he said to her one day, "Why don't you go and concentrate on somebody else?" Here was another comment that suggested that this was someone not with a learning difficulty, but who needed to be able to come alive and really let people know what he was feeling and what he would like to do with his time and his life.

Conductive Education Pilot Study for People with Learning Difficulty

Ellie had talked to the nursing manager of Normansfield about the Conductive Education approach, and said that she was running a group in the hospital based on Conductive Education. One of his colleagues came to him and said "Ellie is just doing a behaviour modification programme", but the manager said "please go and see what she is doing". He returned and said "you are right; she is doing something really special and different".

From then on he gave Ellie great support. It was decided that she should run a formal pilot study investigating this approach in Normansfield, partly funded by the NHS and partly by the Friends of Normansfield.

In 1989 the pilot study was carried out with the aim of comparing the use of the conventional Individual Programme Planning approach with the Conductive Education approach for people with learning difficulties. The Individual Programme Planning approach or Person-Centred Planning approach is widely recognised as a tool for assisting learning disability services to structure and coordinate the support offered to service users.

Support was provided by Val Macey, Manager of the CTAU, Catherine Van De Ven, the District Physiotherapist, Hilary Gooch, the District Occupational Therapist, and the District Psychologist. The results were written up by Val Macey. [11]

Very unfortunately, in the middle of the trial, the nursing manager who had supported the project left to take up another position and was not replaced by someone who might have helped to use the benefits of the project. The outcome of the trial was not discussed by the NHS staff who had supported the project, nor the Friends of the hospital who had helped to fund the project.

Ellie presented the outcome of this pilot project at the World Conference for Physical Therapy, held in the Barbican, London in 1991. The success of the project was that all participants demonstrated improvements in several areas of function which was due to the consistency, continuity and commitment of the multi-disciplinary team. This was over a six-month period.

Creation of Health Record Book and its Benefits

While working in Normansfield, Ellie was involved in treating a girl with spastic quadriplegia, who had to go into Kingston Hospital for surgery on her legs. She was concerned that the daily programme she had set up to help the girl improve her arm function would be neglected while the girl was in hospital.

The programme was aimed at improving her upper arm function and thus giving her some independence. This would have been possible since her surgery did not affect her arms. The staff also might not realise how much the girl could understand, because she had difficulty in verbal communication.

Thus she produced a Health Record Book covering what was done or required throughout all 24 hours of the day, including the arm programme with the aim of assisting the hospital staff in understanding the patient despite her lack of verbal communication. This was the impetus to create the Health Record Book which was positively valuated by one the of students from St George's Medical School who regularly visit Integrated Neurological Services. [See p132]

Monthly Groups for Parkinson's

As a community physiotherapist, Ellie was able to run two monthly groups for people with Parkinson's in Richmond, Twickenham and Roehampton; one in the Keep-Well Elderly Clinic at the Maddison Clinic and one in Kew Baptist Church, using a Conductive Education approach with the support of a clinical psychologist.

Permission to use the Kew Baptist Church premises was first organised through the deacons with the kind assistance of Klara, the wife of the then pastor Robin Dowling. Klara, as a nurse, was very interested in the work that Ellie was doing. The participants appreciated the benefits of the monthly group sessions, but they felt that weekly groups would be more beneficial. Unfortunately, the NHS and the Parkinson's Disease Society were unable to fund such groups on a weekly basis.

Taking the Doctor's Advice – Going Independent

In April 1993 Ellie gave up her job as community physiotherapist and left the NHS. Her GP said *"you don't really have high blood pressure but you will if you continue to work in the NHS, just go and do your work in a different way"*. She left the surgery greatly elated! Thus evolved INS!

"High blood pressure" had a lot to do with the frustration brought about by the lack of follow-up to the £27,000 pedobarograph trial, funded by the Department of Health, and the Normansfield trial, funded by the NHS with the Friends of Normansfield.

Both trials provided interesting results and experience that could be used to help patients, helpers, therapists, professional staff and the service itself; time, expertise, patients' involvement, and money spent to demonstrate possible benefits for stroke patients and those with learning difficulty had been largely wasted.

HOW.....

The Creation of the Charity – Integrated Neurological Services

Pilot Study for People with Parkinson's Showed the Value of the Conductive Education Approach

Meanwhile the two monthly groups, which Ellie had run as a community physiotherapist based at Queen Mary's Hospital, where the participants were people with Parkinson's, formed themselves into a user group called Concern.

On the initiative of one of the members, Miriam Swift, a retired social worker, a money grant was acquired from the Sainsbury Good Neighbour Scheme to help fund a pilot study to demonstrate the value of weekly groups based on Conductive Education.

The pilot study took place in October 1993 at the Maddison Clinic, Church Road, Teddington. The day before it began Ellie met, by chance, an out-of-work social worker, Joan Flint, who came to help the participants write the answers to the pre-project questionnaire, which the participants had helped create. She stayed on to help because she was interested in the Conductive Education approach for neurologically impaired people.

Joan made a huge contribution in continuing to work as a volunteer social worker for eleven years, supporting the groups as part of her work and helping develop what turned out to be the INS charity. She learnt how to help the clients physically by taking part in the groups, e.g. when one fell on the floor during one of her home visits, she was able to give guidance as to how he could get up, thus saving on the need to call an ambulance.

Three therapists – an occupational therapist, speech and language therapist and the psychologist – who had been supporting Ellie's work in the community, assessed the patients before and after the eight group sessions whose holistic programme Ellie had led, based on the Conductive Education approach. The programme was run for an hour.

As a result of the pilot study, the assessors saw some improvements in all three areas: all the participants benefitted in confidence and well-being; there were improvements in facial expression and social skills; and in movement, e.g. putting on a coat. This would not have been the case if the programme had been based solely on physiotherapy.

Most of the participants in the pilot study wished to continue a similar weekly programme and a new Parkinson's group was formed. At first premises were found in a district nurses' base behind the hospital in Teddington. Patients were also being referred, some by GP's who had known Ellie as a community physiotherapist, and some by word of mouth.

Getting Started

In 1994 as a private physiotherapist, Ellie was given a contract with a GP practice in Twickenham – the Wild Practice at St John's Health Centre – to give physiotherapy support for their neurological patients. Patients were visited and treated at home. If appropriate they might be invited to join a group.

In 1994 the Parkinson's group which evolved out of those who had taken part in the Parkinson's Pilot Study moved to Kew Baptist Church by kind permission of the pastor, Steve Gunderson, where Ellie previously had run one of the monthly PD groups while she was a community physiotherapist in the NHS. This group was led by the conductor Judit Szathmary. Two videos were made of her leading the group sessions for teaching purposes. The funds to pay for Judit Szathmary were raised by members of the Concern user group.

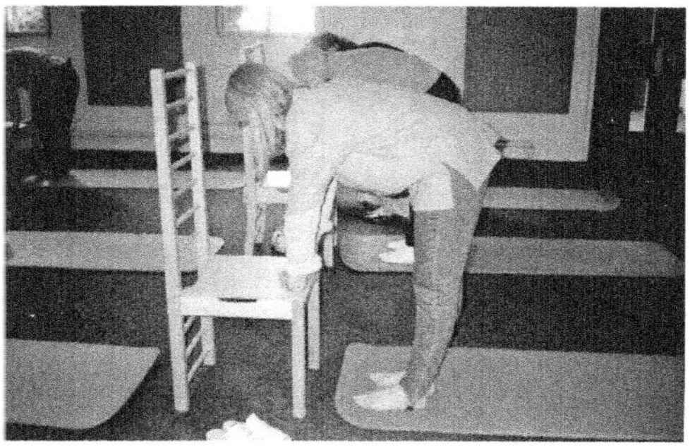

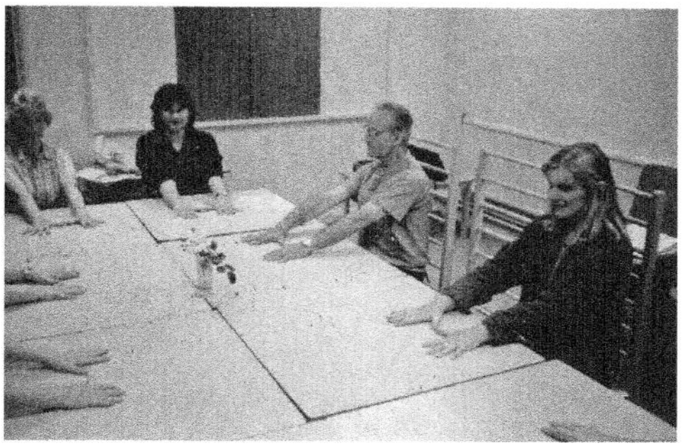

Early Parkinson's Group

Gradually group work was extended from the Parkinson's group to a group for people with MS which took place in the Greenwood Voluntary Care Centre in Hampton Hill, supported by a volunteer social worker, Joan Flint and a physiotherapist, Margot Lucas, who had been the District Physiotherapist at St George's Hospital, Tooting.

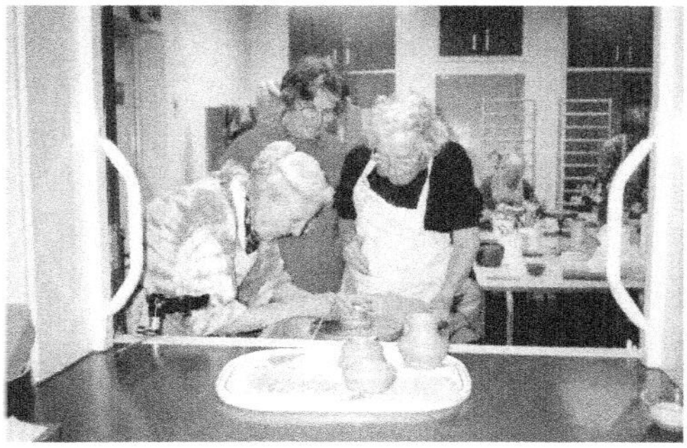

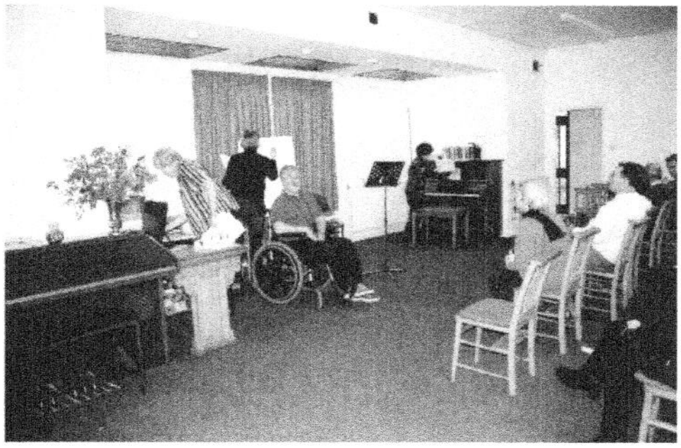

Stroke Group Activities: Pottery and Singing

Later in 1995 a self-help Stroke group was started by Judit Szathmary with Ellie's support in the music room of the home of the composer Andrej Panufnik, who had died a few years before. This was achieved through the kind permission of his wife, Lady Camilla Panufnik, who was a friend of Lady Sheila Hale. Her husband, the Art Historian Sir John Hale, was one of the first members of the group. [See *The Man Who Lost his Language* by Sheila Hale] [12]

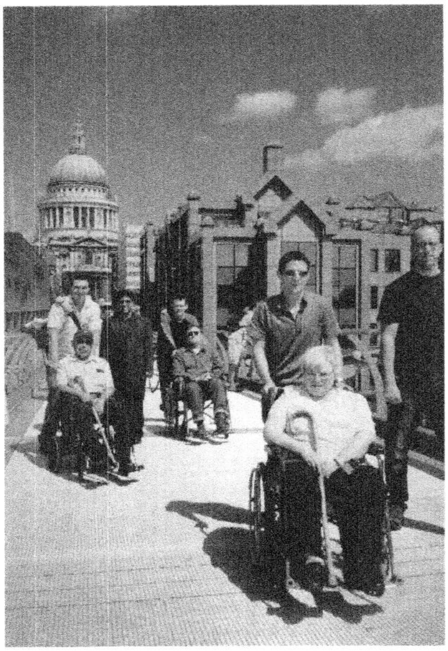
Activities: Outing to St Pauls

When INS became a charity, Sheila became one of the first trustees. The group later moved to Twickenham by kind permission of the warden in the block of flats where two of the patients with a stroke lived.

Further support for the Stroke group was provided by four volunteers; Liz Grove, an occupational therapist; Sue Yorath, a superintendent physiotherapist at the St Helier University Hospital, Carshalton; Wendy Toms, who was a retired ophthalmology business manager with a nursing background; and the social worker, Joan Flint. Judit had to travel from her home in the New Forest.

~~~

Liz Grove had become a carer for her husband and was to play a vital part in the formation of INS. Not only had she been the first Occupational Therapy Officer to the Department of Health, but she had been District Occupational therapist at St George's Hospital, where she had been responsible for the development of the Occupational Therapy Department at the Wolfson Medical Rehabilitation Unit in Wimbledon. There she was involved in working with a multi-disciplinary team where workshops were created to help disabled people return to their occupation or find other more suitable jobs tailored to their changing needs.

With her experience and expertise she was willing to come and work voluntarily full time to help develop the work particularly in support of the carers, develop a Befriending service with the social worker, Joan Flint, and help provide creative pursuits for the groups – art, pottery, music, singing and play reading bringing in expert volunteers in their field.

She was also involved in supervising occupational therapy students on fieldwork placements. In 2002 she was awarded an Honorary Doctorate from Brunel University for her work by influencing and changing professional practice and guiding national policy.

~~~

While waiting for Stroke group participants to arrive Liz arranged for those waiting that they should write down what they had experienced during the week; for those who could no longer write or speak, the family member wrote what he/she had done. They then could read this out when all had arrived to give them more confidence socially.

The group moved to Kew Baptist Church when the morning group "Preparing for the Day" was extended into the afternoon, from 10.30 until 3.30, to give respite to the family carers. In the afternoon the participants took part in different activities organised by Liz such as singing, accompanied by Jan Cunningham, an accompanist and repetiteur for an opera company; carpet bowls led by Liz; art led by Maggie Hughes, the wife of one of participants in the stroke group, who was a trained artist working as an art therapist, with Bridget Boulting, a professional painter; and pottery with Sylvia des Fours, a professional potter, a member of the Craftsman Potters Association. All were volunteers.

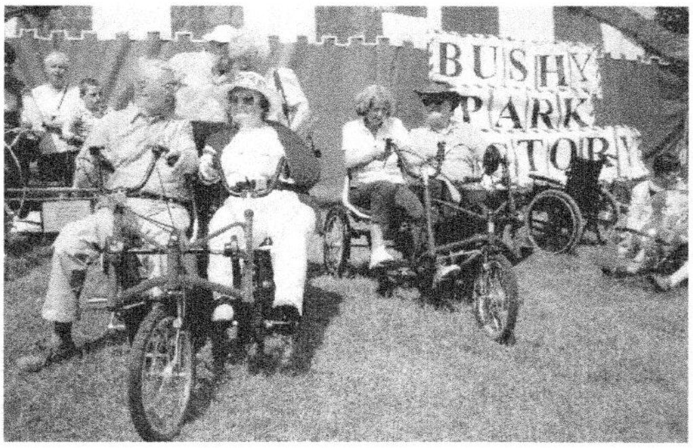

Activities: Companion Cycling

Later Liz organised various outings; to Kew Gardens, to the Wetlands Centre, on the Venturer Boat either towards Richmond or Hampton Court, to the Richmond Theatre and the Orange Tree Theatre. A shopping expedition to Marks & Spencer gave a wonderful opportunity for the participants to choose their own clothes since they had been unable to do their own shopping for a long time and afterwards they got together in the cafe.

Other great outings included a concert in the Festival Hall and a truly memorable outing organised by a young volunteer, when a group of participants, therapists and volunteers drove in a bus to St Paul's Cathedral where they were met by more volunteers from American Express, who kindly helped the patients to be taken to places of their choice – to the Globe Theatre, to HMS Belfast, to St Paul's Cathedral, Festival Hall – all meeting back at St Paul's to be driven back to Kew.

Making Use of a Health Record Book

This time also saw further demonstration of the benefits of having a health record. One of Ellie's clients was in the later stages of Parkinson's, and needed to go into a residential care home for respite care while his wife had a much-needed break. Ellie went to visit the staff prior to his admission, to show them his up-to-date Health Record Book, which contained the information on his past medical history, his medication, and his daily exercise programme to maintain his independence in order to enable him to have a smooth transition at a very difficult time for him and maintain his recent improved mobility.

By doing this it ensured that the staff knew his mobility and strengthening programme and were willing to continue this on a daily basis and they saw the timetable for his daily medication. It was also possible to emphasise that the staff needed to give him his medication at the required time. Without this he might lose his mobility which would make it very awkward for the staff.

It was extremely important for his wife that he did not regress mentally and physically on her return, as the situation was already very difficult for her. His wife was very grateful, after her much-needed break, that he had not deteriorated appreciably and so she could still cope with him living at home.

Registering as a Charity

Liz introduced Professor Pilkington to the emerging team. He was a retired consultant physician who had also worked at St George's Hospital. He was now living in Kew, and he was also a member of the Regional Health Authority, the Area Health Authority and the District Health Authority.

Groups were increasingly run for people with Parkinson's, stroke and MS. Barbara Cook, a retired physiotherapist from the Hospital for Neuro-disability also came to help with the ever-increasing MS group and later with the Stroke group held in Kew Baptist Church.

When it was known that GP Fundholding would cease in 1999 causing the GP practice to be unable to pay for Ellie's work for the practice, Professor Pilkington and Liz were instrumental in encouraging and helping her register the organisation as a charity to provide a way of helping fund the work. A team of potential trustees was formed under the guidance of Professor Pilkington and Integrated Neurological Services was registered as a charity.

Liz knew Baroness Rosalie Wilkins, a previous President of the College of Occupational Therapy, and was able to ask her to became the first Patron of the charity. Later, Liz took over as Chair of the Trustees from Professor Pilkington, a position she held for some years.

The Initial Board of Trustees

Chairman, Professor Thomas Pilkington, Professor Emeritus Medicine
Treasurer, Mr Mervyn Archdall, Business and Financial Advisor
Hon Sec, Mrs Elizabeth Grove, Retired Occupational Therapist, Officer DHSS
Mrs Janet Kingston, Social Worker, Community Mental Health
Mrs Joan Flint, Retired Social Worker
Rev Steven Gunderson, Minister of Kew Baptist Church
Lady Sheila Hale, Family Carer
Mr Richard Jeffries, Retired Director of Social Services
Mrs Margot Lucas, Retired District Physiotherapist
Mrs Susan Yorath, Retired Superintendent Physiotherapist

Co-opted, Ms Susan Ball, Representing the MS users and Director of RAID
Mrs Ann Gould, Representing PD users and carers
Welfare Officer, PD Society, Richmond
Mrs Jill Ritchie, Representing the Stroke Association

The charity was established in recognition of a need for regular, ongoing self-help therapy and support for people with chronic or deteriorating neurological conditions, particularly Parkinson's disease (PD), multiple sclerosis (MS), debilitating stroke or head injury; to develop their self-reliance, enable them to live as independently as possible and thus enhance their quality of life.

The charity also offered support for the family carers. Gradually more and more volunteers joined the charity, working in many different aspects and giving very valuable assistance and expertise.

In 2000, volunteer Belinda Canosa became the first dedicated fundraiser for the charity and gave incredibly valuable work and organised and supported numerous fundraising events. People joined the Friends of INS who came from all walks of life to support the fundraising events and help promote the charity. The demand for INS services grew and larger premises were needed and in 2010 INS moved from Kew Baptist Church to 82, Hampton Road, Twickenham which had a garden. Ann Bond, an occupational therapist and former care manager, who had taken over from Ellie, becoming the first INS Chief Executive, was instrumental in developing the new centre.

The Value of INS' Work

Following a visit to INS and interviews with patients and staff in 2014 Jackie Ashley the famous journalist (and wife of Andrew Marr) with a great interest in neurological matters wrote an article which was published in the Guardian newspaper. Here is an extract.

I've seen the future of Britain's healthcare – and it works

Two therapists identified a desperate need in the community. This is the kind of success story that the NHS must sustain.

Integrated Neurological Services (INS) was set up back in 1999 by Liz Grove and Ellie Kinnear to fill the gaps left by the NHS.

.... In the well-equipped gyms, 10 people are attending a balance class. Beatta, a Parkinson's patient, is losing her balance, but wants to show her fellow patients how yoga has helped her. John has agreed with Frank to swap skills – John will teach Frank guitar-playing, while Frank will help John on the computer. Other patients take part in memory classes, cooking skills and speech therapy.

.... When you are hit with a long-term medical condition your life – and your family's life – changes totally. But the charity aims to help you adapt, to share experiences with people suffering from the same conditions and to learn skills that may enable you to live a fulfilling life, maybe following a different pathway.

The two key words from all staff are "patient-centred". Everyone is individually assessed to help them through the system. That can be anything from finding clinical help, medication, physical therapy, emotional support, housing support and help for the carers too.

The patients I met felt valued, supported and empowered. One stroke survivor had found that Nordic walking (with ski poles) helped his movement and fitness, so the team persuaded him to lead a group in Nordic walking once a week.

.... Parkinson's, multiple sclerosis and stroke are the diseases we are increasingly suffering from, as the medical advances in heart disease and cancer mean that we live longer. Physical therapy, just as much as drugs, can help with recovery from stroke and with delaying the onset of symptoms from Parkinson's and multiple sclerosis.

.... how can this small but brilliant organisation provide a national model?

Extract from article by Jackie Ashley published in *The Guardian*, June 2014

Education – INS Involvement with St George's Medical School

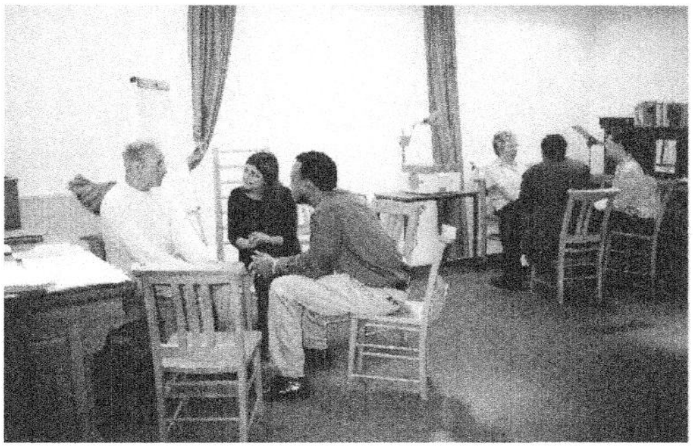

St George's Medical Students Talking with Clients

INS provides a unique educational programme for medical students from St George's Medical School, focusing on the consequences of neurological conditions.

In a typical year dozens of INS clients and carers will help INS provide 20 or so sessions to over 300 medical students to help them understand the impact of living with a neurological condition. The students hear the patient and carer experience in small interactive workshops.

Margot Turner, Senior Lecturer in Diversity and Medical Education at St George's Medical School says:

"St George's Medical School and INS have been working together for about 20 years now. Our students have been able to learn so much about how neurological conditions effects both patients and families. The student feedback has always been so positive both from the medical students and the INS participants.

This year we were afraid they wouldn't be able to go ahead because of COVID. I should have known better, of course INS staff, users and families worked very hard and have been able to recreate the visits virtually and the students have been so pleased that the visits were able to go ahead and they were able talk to people and learn from everyone at INS."

Quotes from medical students include: *"Really inspiring session, talking to patients was fantastic." "Very informative discussions with patients, I learnt a lot."*

Earlier on two medical students were inspired to carry out research for INS. One was a survey to evaluate the effectiveness of INS with clinical measurements of clinical progress in relation to their ability to maintain or improve activities of daily living and to evaluate INS' therapeutic efficacy compared to the few available benchmarks.

The survey found that after nine months treatment, INS reported measurable improvements in three quarters of all stroke patients, half of the Parkinson's patients and one third of MS patients. This is corroborated by other stroke research but also supports research evidence which suggests that improvements can be achieved with continued therapy input for people with Parkinson's and MS.

The other was a survey of all INS carers. The objective of this study was to assist INS in measuring the benefits of the service to carers and to aid future planning by identifying new services that would be of value to the carers. This was a very useful exercise which demonstrated the value of support given to carers by INS and also provided a number of new ideas on how the service could be expanded and developed. Many of the ideas were included in the INS strategic plan.

Placements

Additionally, INS takes undergraduate health and social care professionals on clinical placements and recently supported four students studying courses in physiotherapy, occupational and speech and language therapy on eight and four-week placements.

My Group – A Doctor Speaks

This is by Ellie's GP

~~~~~

"You've got Parkinson's syndrome; this could be caused by any number of neurodegenerative disorders". There followed a list of possible diagnoses varying from the dire to the progressively lethal and then I was out in the
~~~~~

corridor with a vague promise of a 10-minute appointment in four months' time, and my resolve to think positively draining away.

No mention of a physiotherapist, Parkinson's disease nurse or the Parkinson's Disease Society, perhaps as a GP I was expected to know how to cope with the ebbing of my future plans.

Fortuitously, one of my patients is a neurophysiotherapist, convinced of the value of holistic care and self-help for chronic neurological conditions. She was supportive and encouraging when I phoned her, and visited me and my husband at home two days later.

"We will meet this challenge together; you are very welcome to the weekly group."

In our group, personalities and individuality shine through and we almost forget our disease. James has lived in a religious community for 50 years and has calmly adapted to the disease, attending our group despite now living 30 miles away and being an important carer for a member of the community who has cancer. Vanessa uses every ounce of energy and won't slow down; she is our drug expert as she has experienced the effects and side effects of virtually every' available drug. She keeps us up to date with research and longs for a cure, hating the disease and the limitations it is putting on her life.

Peter paints and writes poetry despite the horrible side effects of apomorphine, he never moans, except the time he asked for any new ideas to help constipation. Carol finds walking difficult but she has just returned from a successful cycling holiday in France and is planning the next one despite having had PD for 10 years. Ann is the joker, though most of her stories must be censored, and as long as he doesn't freeze, and can find the time amongst all his other activities Graham takes wonderful photos.

We meet with our physiotherapist, occupational therapist and social worker, and over coffee we share events, hopes and fears of the previous week. Then we exercise, stretch and practise coordination, balance and relaxation, all relating to daily activities. Workshops sometimes follow the group, play readings to help us articulate and project our voices, mindful acting to help with self-expression. Singing and painting workshops, are planned.

We are all enriched by this session, and gain infinitely more than can ever be achieved in a routine out-patient appointment, where our capacity and inclination to express our anxieties and perspectives of our condition are limited by time, the daunting environment and difficulties with speech.

We have many visitors, students, mainly physio and OT, members of the-PDS, Parkinson's disease nurses from overseas, complementary therapists, carers and other voluntary workers. So much can be shared and discovered by both patients and a range of professionals, but neither medical students, GPs, nor hospital doctors have accepted our invitation to attend and there is no NHS funding.

Graham is always depressed by his hospital appointment, when he may see different doctors of different experience, some of who have never seen him before and will not be there the next time. He is shy and self-conscious and cannot easily articulate his views and frustrations and is more comfortable in the written word. This is what he composed and recited at one of our meetings, and he speaks for us all.

IT TAKES A LITTLE LONGER NOW

It takes a little longer now
To get the small things done.
The things that used to do themselves
Need battles to be won.

It takes longer now to fit a plug,
The screw's fall to the floor
And as you bend to pick them up,
They roll away some more.

It takes longer now to shave and dress,
To put on socks and shoes,
These chores are so frustrating
You really get the blues.

It takes a little longer now
To organise your life,
To recognise the problems
That can strain a man and wife.

It takes a little longer now
So please give us some time
This crazy thing called Parkinson

Has grabbed us in our prime.

It takes a little longer now
I really do my best,
Please show some understanding
I'll try to do the rest.

It takes a little longer now
To get out of a freeze
To get your legs to hold you up
Sod Parkinson's disease

Stop moaning now, you can't do much
To change the state of play,
There's lots of people worse than you,
A cure might come your way.

[The above is from an article for the *British Medical Journal,* but not published.]

How the Diagnosis Can Affect the Person

Two years after her diagnosis Ellie's doctor was unable to continue her work as a GP. Ellie asked her if she could help with the medical students. For this she drew up the following:

Response of a GP to a diagnosis that she had Parkinson's disease

Breaking Bad News ***Doctor's perception (me)***	**Breaking Bad News** ***Patient's perception (me)***
Listen well Empathy Part of the job	Life devastating event Changes everything
Doctor-patient relationship is all Good doctor can cope alone	Need a friend/nurse/therapist present Need more time, very happy to talk to a nurse
Lots of information is good	Forget most of what is said
Poor you	I can't work, I'll be in a home by the time I'm 60

But it's not cancer, it's not fatal	
Be positive, enjoy yourself	Depression, shock, denial
Nothing needs to be done now See you in four months	Desperate for support Named person Phone numbers self-help group
Follow up Appointments ***Doctor (me)***	**Follow up Appointments** ***Patient(me)***
It's good practice to always examine the patient	I want my agenda followed; my concerns addressed
I'll adjust the drugs	Why am I having another neurological examination? My reflexes might be normal, but there are lots of symptoms that worry me There must be more to my treatment than drugs
I'll see you again soon	
Prescribing *Doctor (me)*	**Prescribing** *Patient(me)*
Take one 3 times a day	How do I take them? What exactly?
All drugs have side effects, you might have a little nausea, try them and see	I can't cope with side effects; I can't cope with feeling even iller
Give lots of information	Thanks for the information, but it is the wrong information
Listen to the patient	Please hear my concerns Let me see the agenda

NOTES AND REFERENCES

[1] She was a founder member of the Association of Chartered Physiotherapists in Neurology (ACPIN), which evolved from the Hemiplegic Interest Group.

[2] This led Ellie to look for an opportunity to be involved with the education of medical students. Medical students from St George's Medical School, Tooting, first came to visit the INS charity in 2002 and continue to do so to the present day.

[3] In 1991 Ester was given a doctorate in Education from Queen Margaret's College at Edinburgh University for her work in bringing this Conductive Education approach out of Hungary and introducing it to different parts of the world.

[4] Hong Kong Physiotherapy Journal, Vol. 8. 1986, Special Issue CONDUCTIVE EDUCATION

[5] E. A. Bilodeau, *Principles of Skill Acquisition*, Academic Press, 1969

[6] Using objective inter-related, reliably-tested measurements. A Physical Assessment for Stroke Patients, Physiotherapy, 1982, 68, no4, pp109-113

[7] F. B. Gibberd, N. G. R. Page, K. M. Spencer, E. Kinnear, J. B. Hawksworth, *Controlled trial of physiotherapy and occupational therapy for Parkinson's disease*, British Medical Journal, 1981, Vol. 282, 1196 https://www.bmj.com/content/282/6271/1196.1

[8] W. J. Perkins, *A video aid to assessment and retraining of standing balance, Chapter 5, High Technology Aids for the Disabled,* Butterworth-Heinemann, 1983

M. Lord, E. Kinnear, D. M. Smith, *Video aid to rehabilitation of standing balance,* Medical & Biological Engineering & Computing (MBEC), 1982, 20, pp281-285 https://link.springer.com/article/10.1007/BF02442793

Video aid to rehabilitation of standing balance in Hemiparesis, 7th International Symposium on External Control of Human Extremities, pp177-187, at conference Advances in External Control of Human Extremities, in Belgrade, 1981

[9] *Long-term management of Parkinson's Disease*, Physiotherapy Journal, July 1986, Vol. 72, no7

[10] L. Eve, E. Kinnear, *Does the Wheelchair Fit?* Physiotherapy Journal, 1989, Vol. 75, no2

https://www.physiotherapyjournal.com/article/S0031-9406(10)62710-1/fulltext

[11] The review of a pilot project at Normansfield Hospital using the principles of Conductive Education by V. Macey, Head Occupational Therapist Manager of CTAU and the comments of the two assistants in the Conductive Education programme

[12] Sheila Hale, *The Man Who Lost his Language*, Allen Lane, 2002

~~~~~
~~~~~

Appendix 1
Basic Morning Programme for any Neurological Condition to Prepare for the Day

From a Physiotherapy and Physiological Viewpoint

Aim - to improve or maintain good posture, range of movement, and strength, to achieve maximum independence and quality of life.

The programme would be supervised by a physiotherapist or a carer who had been taught how to support the patient with the appropriate programme.

LYING

[Physio] The starting position for the day after the person has woken up. Here gravity is eliminated; the programme in this position requires no balance and is therefore safe for the person to practise the programme independently.

[Physiological] This programme may use the neuroplasticity of the nervous system to reinforce the motor control circuitry for future movements. The same wiring is required for movements that are used in other postures.

I lie well

[Physio] The person is asked to say the action in the first person singular so that ownership of the movement is achieved. To repeat the action will help memory, speech and volume.

[Physiological] By using another input, i.e. speech – which provides both a motor and an auditory input for planning in the pre-motor and supplementary motor cortex – the circuitry is strengthened by further synaptic inputs onto the final motor neurone and hence it's membrane potential will be closer to the threshold level for an action potential which is needed for the muscle to work.

Head in the middle

[Physio] Symmetry is vital for balance

[Physiological] Head control is the fundamental control for all movements. The head position "sets" the normal central position of the body as the central specialised sensory organ of balance which lies in the inner ear. The receptors in this organ, the vestibular apparatus, quickly adapt and can resist the "norm" position which is used as a reference centre for all following movements based on the body position. It has a key role in balance... hence if the "norm" is altered then the balance will be compromised and difficult to maintain. Symmetry uses the forces of gravity for balance, if the body weight falls directly through the central line there will be less energy required to control balance, however if the body is outside the centre then movements will continually be required to prevent falling as the force of gravity will tend to pull the body further out of alignment.

Shoulders level

[Physio] Symmetry vital for balance

[Physiological] Similarly, the symmetrical position is critical for future movements. It creates a base line map on which the motor control system can write the programmes for movement

Back straight, hips straight, knees straight

[Physio] If the person is upright with the above then the centre of gravity will lie in the correct position for maximum stability in standing.

[Physiological] As above it is essential to lay down the correct base line starting position; or map of where each body segment is in relation to each other.

Arms by my sides, fingers stretched, thumb out

[Physio] This is the normal positions of the arms in standing so that no muscle group is working more than another with the hands relaxed.

Toes up (preparation for standing)

[Physio] To have the toes up allows for good weightbearing through the heels for stability of the person in standing

[Physiological] Doing exercises to bring the toes up, again reinforces the neural circuits for this movement that is essential to be able to stand and walk, but also strengthens the muscles required to shift the toes off the ground in walking.

Take a deep breath in and a long breath out

Put your hands on either side of your rib cage, feel the ribs pushing out as you breathe in, feel the ribs sink down as you breathe out.

Repeat feeling your diaphragm expanding all round your waist and relax breathing out, realising that your diaphragm is sinking down, repeat breathing in to the count of four, breath out to the count of six a few times

[Physio] This is to restore health, vitality and energy.

[Physiological] Breathing slowly and deeply ensures adequate ventilation for future movements by providing adequate oxygen for the cells to provide energy for the movements and therefore function. It allows the whole lungs to be inflated and hence more force for expiration and cough to remove secretions.

I turn my head to the right/left

[Physio] This is important to be able to see people or objects as in driving.

I tuck my chin in and lift my head to look at my right/left toes and down

[Physio] This engages the abdominal muscles to help the person have core control

[Physiological] Movements using neck muscles are particularly important not only for functional activities, but also because of the high number of muscle receptors in the neck which are responsible for the brain to interpret where the head is in relation to other body segments and are used to give feedback control during standing and moving.

I lift my arms up (right/left, both) and breathe in, I left my arms down and breathe out

[Physio] To encourage full elevation of the arms with expansion of the ribs.

[Physiological] This will ensure good ventilation volume and full range of movement of the shoulder joint. Practising the movement in lying allows the pathways for movement control to be stored in memory.

I clasp my hands together

[Physio] This brings the hands into midline for symmetry and allows the stronger hand to assist the weaker hand to be mobilised and useful thus avoiding neglect of the weaker hand.

[Physiological] Clasping hands together will also stimulate sensory receptors which will reinforce the central position and the movement pathway.

I lift my hands to the ceiling and down

[Physio] This helps to mobilise the shoulders into elevation.

I lift my hands above my head to touch the wall and down

[Physio] This helps to achieve full mobilisation of the shoulder and gives a goal for the person to reach when positioned appropriately.

I lift my hands behind my neck

[Physio] This brings the arms into full external rotation into a position where the person has to wash their neck, comb their hair and put their collar into the correct position. It also allows the person to put in their earrings.

I bring my elbows together and apart

[Physio] This mobilises the shoulders into external and internal rotation to help with dressing and a variety of tasks.

I bring my hands down

[Physio] Ready to start the next task.

I put my hands on my chin and down

I put my hands on my nose and down

I put my hands on my forehead and down

I put my hands on top of my head and down

[Physio] These movements are helping to mobilise the shoulders and the elbows in midline.

I put my hands on my right/left shoulder

I put my hands on my right/left ear

[Physio] These movements are to bring the arms into rotation.

I turn my hands inside out

[Physio] This is to achieve full elbow, wrist and finger extension.

I lift my hands above my head

[Physio] This is to achieve full shoulder elevation with full elbow, wrist and finger extension which is a position of normal stretch e.g. athletes.

These tasks can be repeated in sitting and should be encouraged until the person is able to do them with ease.

[Physiological] All the above exercises will reinforce the motor pathways to be stored in motor memory, which can be utilized in activities of daily living. It is practising elements of movement that will be part of whole movement strategies for tasks – function for motor learning.

I put my hands on my shoulders. I push my elbows into the bed, pull my shoulder blades together and push my head into the pillow, hold and relax

[Physio] This helps to extend the upper back which is important for good posture and balance.

I lie straight

[Physio] This is a preparation for standing with symmetry for balance.

I bend my right /left leg and put my right/left foot on the bed

I straighten my leg

[Physio] This is to encourage flexion at the hip with the foot flat to encourage weightbearing on the heel which is a preparation for walking.

I clasp my right/left knee to my chest and down

[Physio] This will encourage the hands to be engaged by clasping the hands together for symmetry – increased hip and knee flexion, by bringing the head towards the knee, the abdominal muscles will be engaged to increase core control.

I put both feet flat on the bed with knees bent

[Physio] This will achieve symmetry with a short lever.

I swing my knees to the right/left and look to the left/right

[Physio] Through rotation at the hips, this will increase trunk control and allow stretching of the trunk and the neck.

I bring my hips to mid line

[Physio] For symmetry and to prepare for the next task.

I breath in, I breath out, I pull my tummy in and lift my hips up, hold and relax (Pilates)

[Physio] This is to gain core control and hip extension which is a preparation for standing and walking.

[Physiological] In addition to the neural pathway benefits of these exercises the core muscles are important for balance control and therefore exercises are essential to increase their strength.

I straighten my legs

I roll to the right; I look to the right; I bring my left arm over to the right and roll over

[Physio] This is a preparation for getting out of bed or being able to alter position when in bed, giving independence for greater comfort.

I swing my legs over the side, I lift my head, I push on my right elbow and hand and sit up (repeat on the other side)

[Physio] This engages the whole body and should be practised coming out of bed towards the weaker side to strengthen the muscles and weighbearing on that arm.

I sit straight , feet on the floor, hands on my knees or flat on the bed to stretch my fingers

[Physio] This enables weightbearing through the heels for stability, back straight for standing straight and hands flat on the bed to get weightbearing on the heel of the hands to have fingers straight and the wrist in extension, stimulating the shoulder muscles, the extensors of the elbow and wrists to counteract the effect of spasticity, which causes the wrist and the fingers to bend.

[Physiological] These exercises will not only provide the neural pathways for functional tasks which are prerequisites for rolling and sitting but will also provide additional input through the sensory receptors which will alter the motor neurone membrane potential so that the central motor control system will require less energy. The sensory receptors lie in the joints, muscles and tendons as well as pressure and touch receptors in the skin. By stimulating the extensors the flexor group of muscles in the upper limb will be reciprocally inhibited, hence reducing the possibility of spasticity.

Given below are the comments of a Care Manager on observing the lying programme in action.

.... I was very pleased to have a first-hand opportunity to be able to observe the two carers working on the lying programme. I could see that it was quite safe for the carers to do this with close support and that there were no Health and Safety issues. I noted too that the carers get an enormous amount of satisfaction from assisting her with the exercises. This proved to me that giving her time, and the physical input not only gave her a lot of self-esteem and dignity in trying to do even the smallest movement by herself, but the carers obviously gained a huge amount of job satisfaction.

Obviously, the main aim of the programme is to help keep people as strong and mobile as possible and for as long as possible. I can see that this would also have a huge impact on their self-worth and self-image. I could see that even the client's speech had improved due to repeating the phrases spoken by the carers. Wonderful.

I cannot praise this programme enough; I feel it should be implemented with anyone who has physical limitations for whatever reasons. It is obviously working for my service user, and I cannot thank you enough on her behalf.

Signed Care Manager

SITTING

[Physio] As preparation for standing up and walking.

I put my hands on my knees

[Physio] To encourage balance in sitting.

I push my hands down to touch my ankles

[Physio] This is to familiarise the person with bringing the head forwards which is essential for standing up. It increases the mobility and strength of the hips and the spine.

[Physiological] The balance control system is challenged by bringing the body weight forward and the vestibular system in the head and the muscle spindles in the neck will be excited to provide feedback to the motor control system to regain balance. Not only will this exercise increase strength in the postural muscles, but will also set the central alignment from the feedback in the muscles and joints about the starting position for balance control.

I sit up straight (preparation for standing)

I put my hands flat on the bed (assistance may need to be given by asking the person) I clasp my hands together, I turn my hands inside out, I put my left hand (the weaker hand) on the bed, I separate my hands, I put my right hand down on the right side.

[Physio] This causes the arms to go into some abduction with weightbearing on the heel of the hands to strengthen the arms.

I lean sideways to put my right/left elbow on the bed, push down on the hand and sit up

[Physio] This increases the strength of the arms with increasing mobility and strength of the trunk side flexors muscles. Support may be needed to be given on the back of the hand to fix the hand onto the bed when pushing up on the weaker side.

I push my feet forwards and back

I bring my right/left foot out to the side and in

[Physio] This prepares for placing the feet in the correct position for standing up with the feet slightly apart, level and back near the bed.

[Physiological] Foot placement with steps will provide the motor memory with the correct pathway for an initial step i.e. which muscles need to be activated, when and by how much i.e. it 'writes' a programme for the whole sequence which can then be incorporated into walking without each separate action being controlled independently for coordination.

I lift my right/left foot up and down, marking time 1/2

[Physio] By counting, this increases hip flexion and strengthens the legs and allows the action to be done for longer using rhythm (and song)

[Physiological] By adding the time element, a fuller programme is 'written' into motor memory, now with fuller movements of hips flexion muscles. There is an inherent rhythmicity within this basic circuit at spinal cord level and this can be switched on by the addition of a sensory input e.g. auditory beat so the movement becomes more automatic and so requires less energy.

I bring my feet back (heels on the floor) I lean forwards and stand up

[Physio] By asking the person to repeat the action verbally they will be helped to remember the sequence.

The aim is for the person to do those actions with as little assistance as possible and to rely on the therapist as little as possible for they are present during the day for such a short time. The actions need to be repeated until the actions can be carried out independently with some speed and spontaneity.

STANDING

I stand straight

I stand well - feet level slightly apart, head in the middle, back straight, hips straight, knees straight, hands by my sides

[Physiological] The speech input also acts as additional synaptic input onto the motor neurones, both in memory and at the sensory/motor planning level.

As weight goes through the feet, the pressure receptors and the proprioceptors for the whole limb will be acting on the motor neurone through the feedback/feedforward pathways.

Weight through all the lower limb and trunk muscles, joints, tendons and pressure receptors will not only reinforce the balance control circuitry in memory, but also via direct connections at the spinal motor neurone level.

At this stage other sensory input is equally important i.e. visual – a mirror to continually consciously monitor symmetry for balance. This will then enhance the control pathways into memory, and balance can be restored as automatic without full conscious level and hence be less energy dependent.

I turn to the right/left, I look straight forwards

[Physio] To practise balancing while moving.

I step forward with my stronger leg and back

[Physio] To increase weightbearing on the weaker leg and hip extension.

I step out to the side with my stronger leg

[Physio] To increase weightbearing on the weaker leg with abduction.

I clasp my hands together

[Physio] To engage both hands for symmetry and avoid neglect of the weaker hand which may have reduced sensation.

I lift my hands to shoulder height and down

[Physio] To increase balance awareness with movement away from the body's centre of gravity.

I lift my hands to my mouth and down

[Physio] By moving the hands to a variety of positions this will increase the ability to balance.

I put my hands down by my sides

[Physio] By returning to the starting position this will bring the body into balance ready for the next task.

[Physiological] The above exercises all practise the prerequisites for balance and then movement. They will reinforce the necessary pathways for control mechanisms by stimulating sensory receptors to enable the higher centres to map the position of stability and how to resolve any diversions. They will also strengthen the muscles required to weightbear through a compromised limb and then allow an independent step to be taken.

Turning movements are programmed in the brain stem level, controlled primarily by the basal ganglia group of neurones before they can be used by the primary motor control centres to be incorporated into full movement. Hence it is critical to relearn the programme and reinforce circuitry before complex full movements are undertaken.

Dr Marian Huett, Lecturer in Physiology at King's College Medical School

Eleanor Kinnear, Physiotherapist, member of ACPIN

~~~~~
~~~~~

Appendix 2
Normal Positions to Support Muscles & Joints

This Appendix shows photographs of normal positions that may be taken up throughout the day, demonstrating weightbearing and stretching that should be encouraged for anyone with a neurological condition.

These positions help prevent tightness/spasticity of muscles and help stimulate the muscles around the shoulder, elbow and wrist and fingers. It also helps to prevent pain around the shoulder and arm due to strain/stress of the unsupported weight of the arm on the structures around the shoulder.

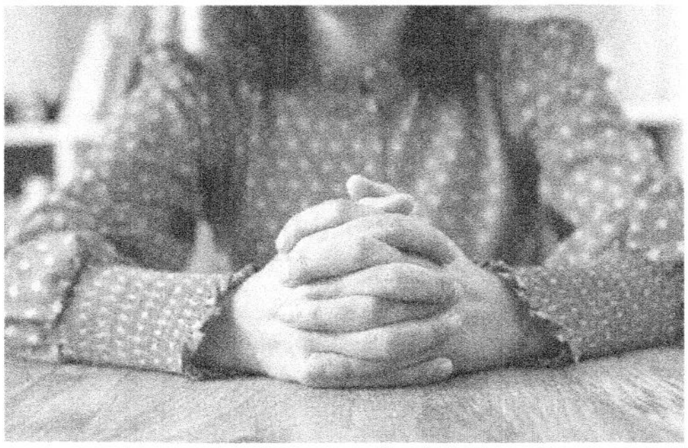

1. The arms weightbearing on the table with clasped hands in midline leaning on the table – stretching the spaces between the fingers

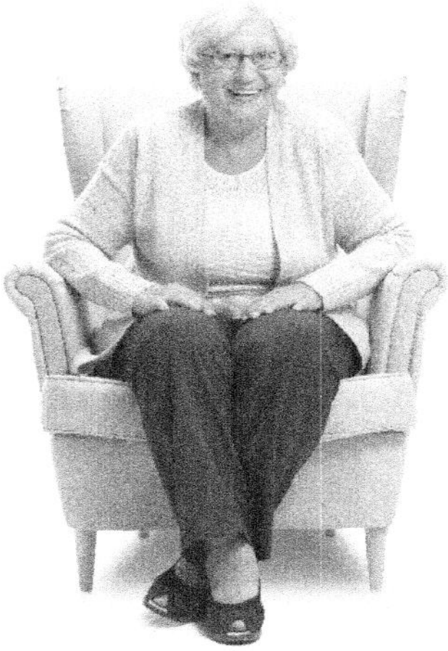

2. Lady sitting symmetrically with both elbows resting on the arms of the chair with the hands and fingers stretched.

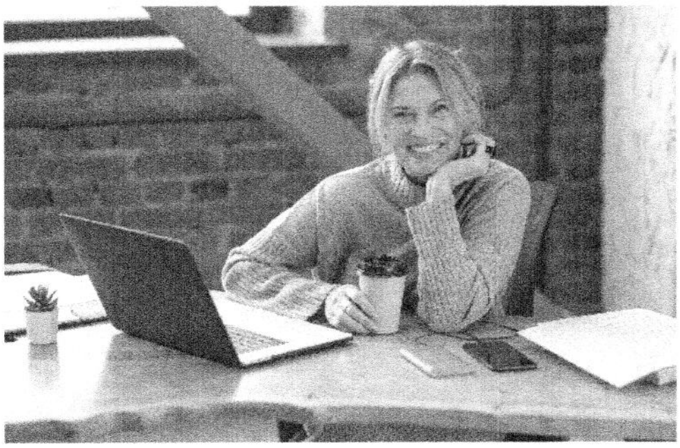

3. Girl leaning her right forearm on the table with her left elbow leaning on the table with the left wrist stretched.

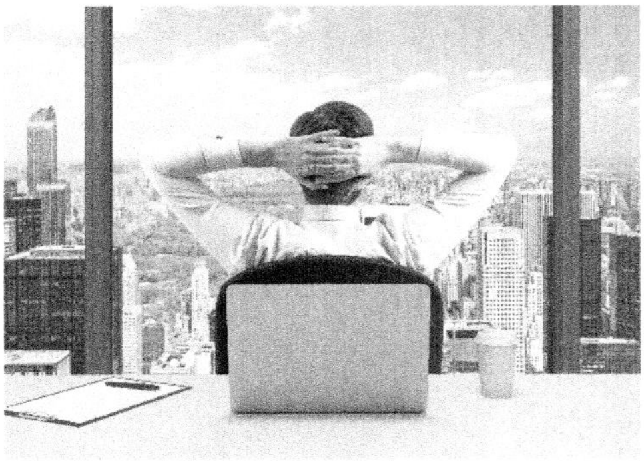

4. Man sitting on a chair with hands clasped, stretching his shoulders and fingers behind his neck.

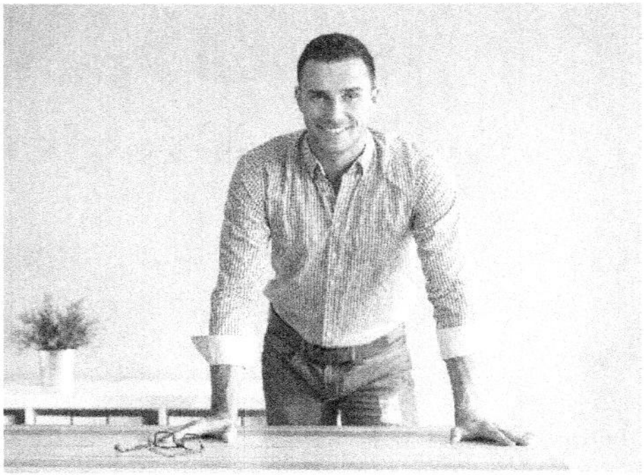

5. Man standing weightbearing both hands flat on the table, stretching both wrists and his elbows.

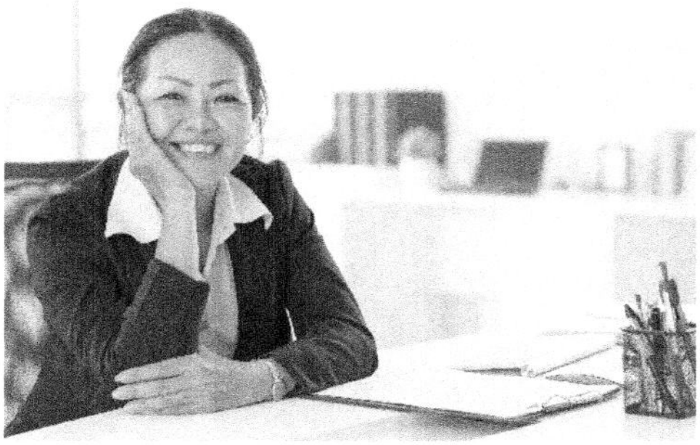

6. Lady weightbearing on her right elbow and left forearm with her right hand stretched over her cheek.

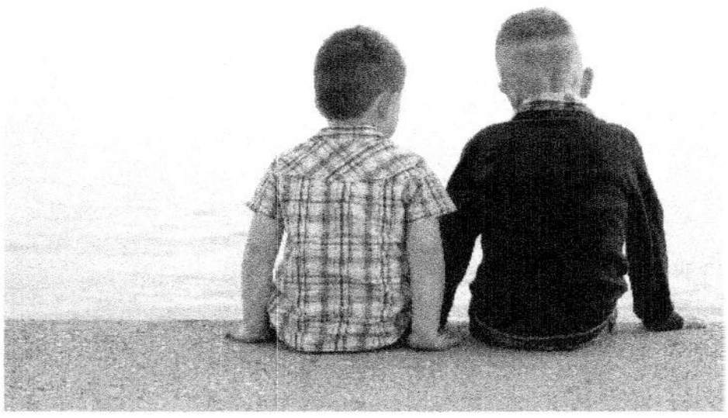

7. Two children weightbearing on both hands, with wrists and elbows stretched.

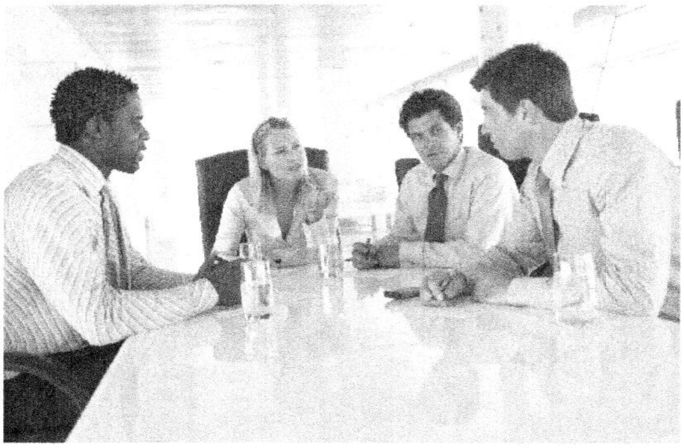

8. A group of people chatting round a table leaning on their forearms in a variety of positions of weightbearing.

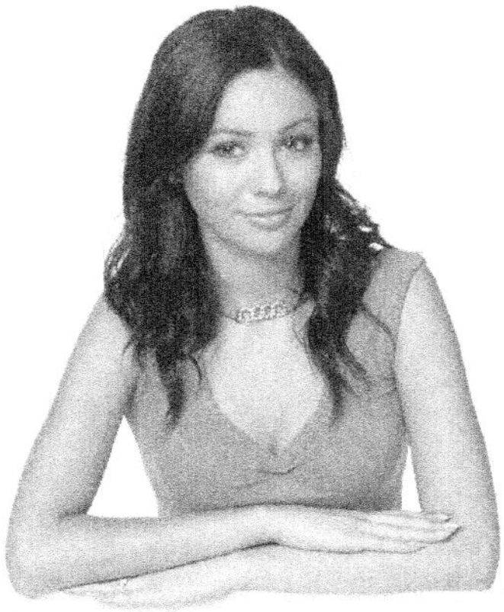

9. Girl leaning on both arms symmetrically with both hands and fingers stretched.

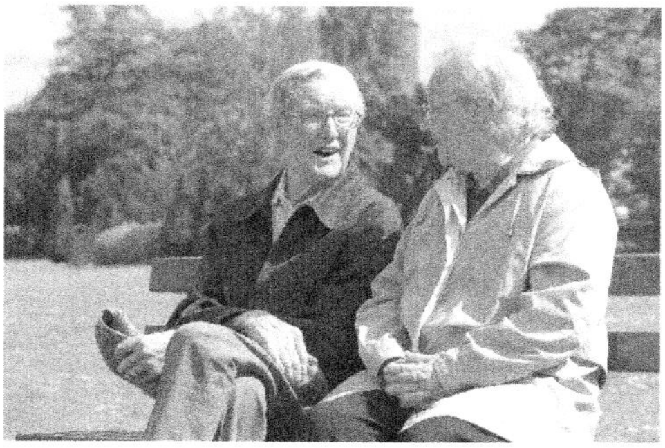

10. A couple sitting chatting on a bench with the lady sitting with her hands clasped in midline and the man with his arms crossed relaxing his hands leaning on his thigh.

Appendix 3
Use of a Ladder Chair to Rehabilitate Walking

Section 1 – Aim: To mobilise the hands before placing them on the appropriate rung of the ladder

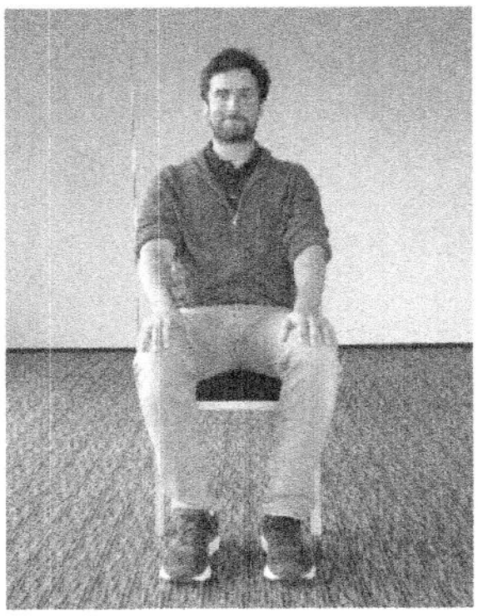

1 Sitting well with hands flat on the knees

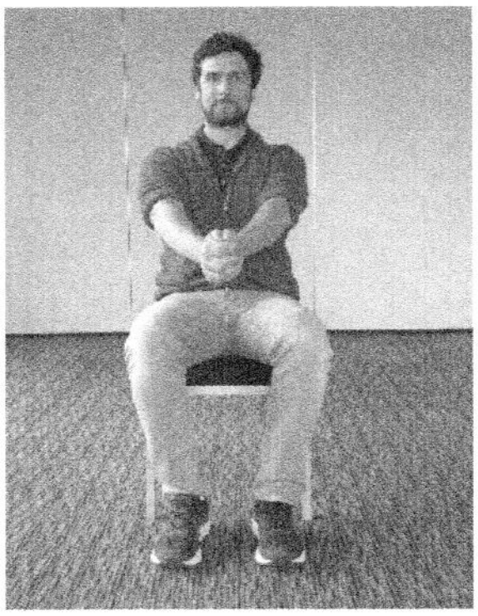

2 Clasping hands together

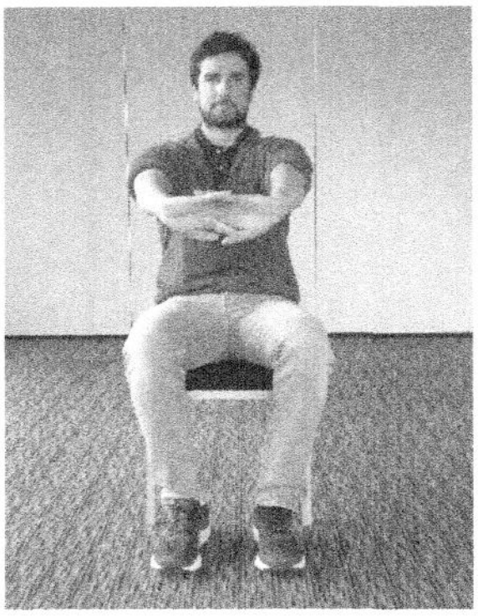

3 Turning hands inside out to stretch the wrists

Section 2 – Aim: To go from sitting to standing with hands clasped for symmetry and have equal weight on both legs for good balance

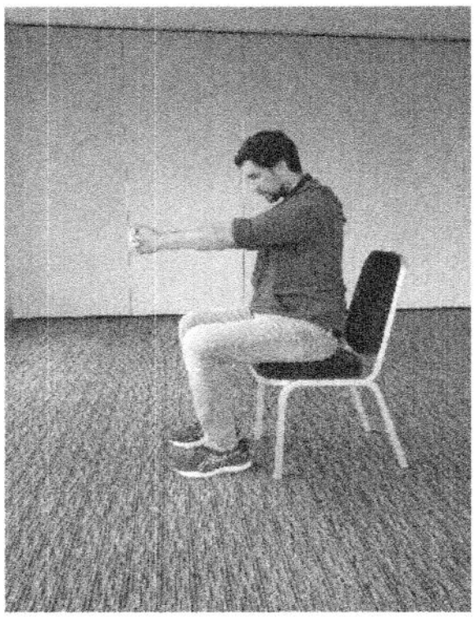

4 Clasped hands raised

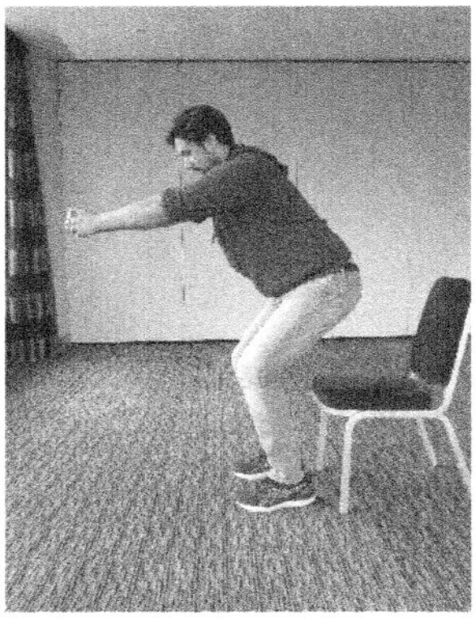

5 Pushing head and hands over the feet to stand up

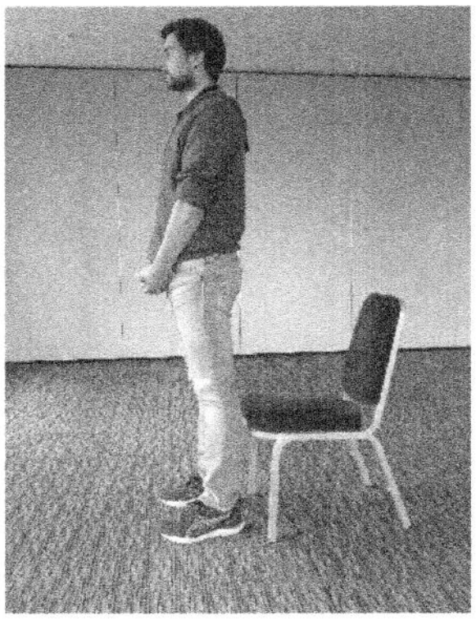

6 Standing straight

Section 3 – Aim: To put hands on the rung of the chair

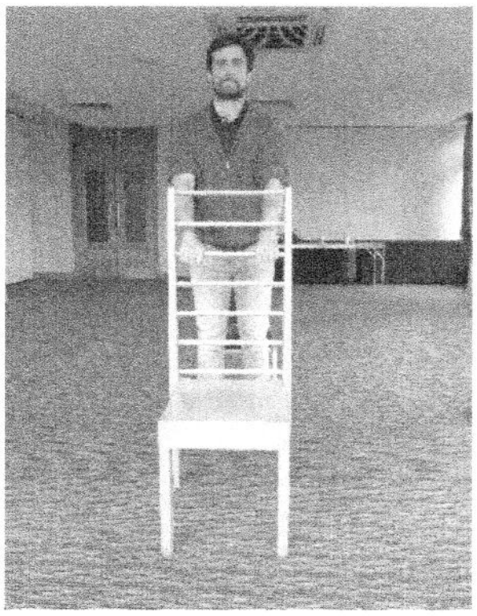

7 Hands can independently grasp the rung

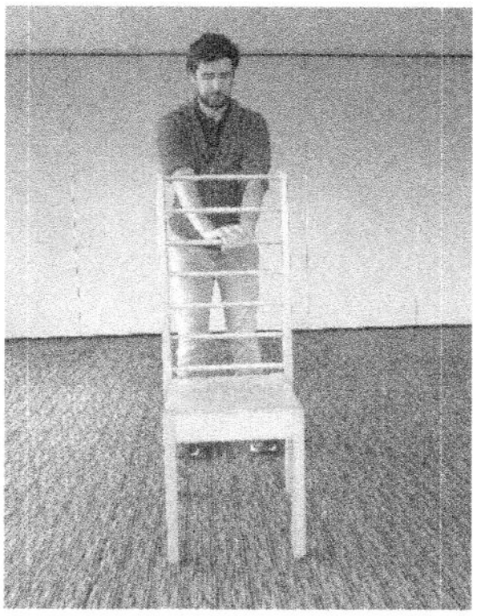

8 Assistance of hands clasped, turning inside out for the stronger hand to fix the weaker hand onto the middle of the rung

Section 4 – Aim: Walking by pushing the chair forwards over a stable four-legged base with goal of walking with a rhythm – step, push, step, push; progressing to counting one, two; one, two

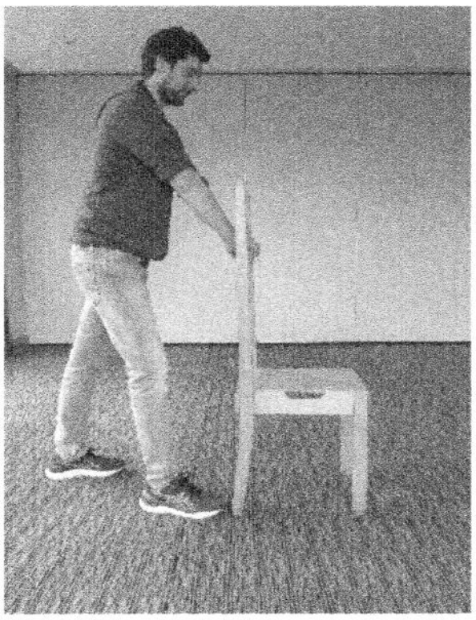

9 Stepping forward with the right foot

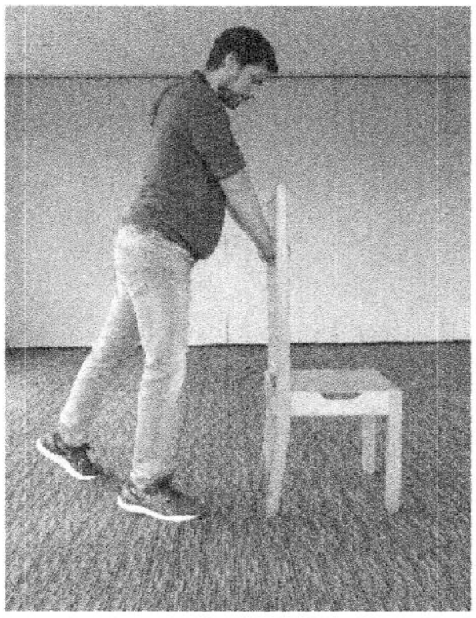

10 Pushing the chair forwards, right hip extension

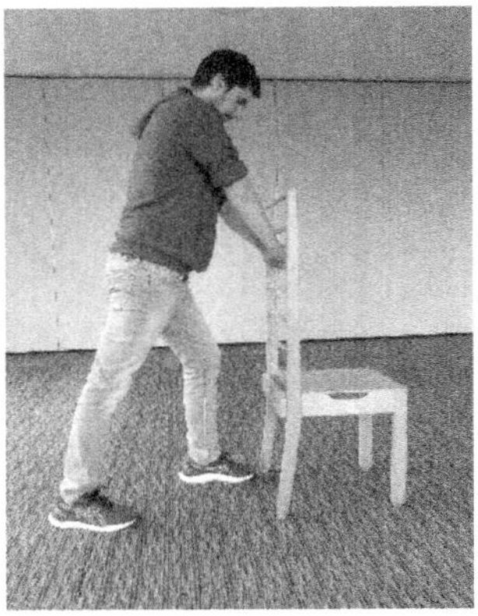

11 Stepping forward with the left foot

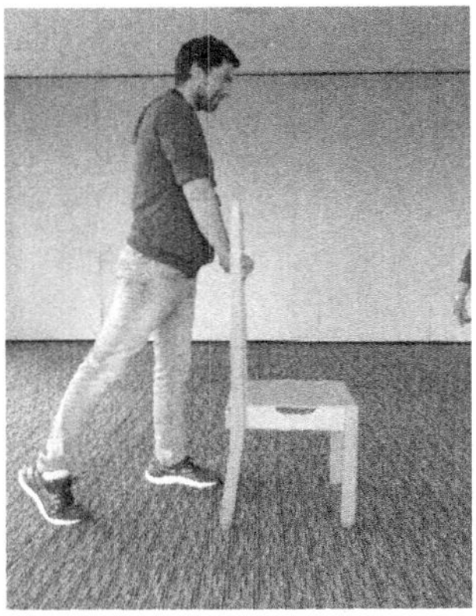

12 Left hip extension

Section 5 – Aim: Mobilising the affected hip and ankle

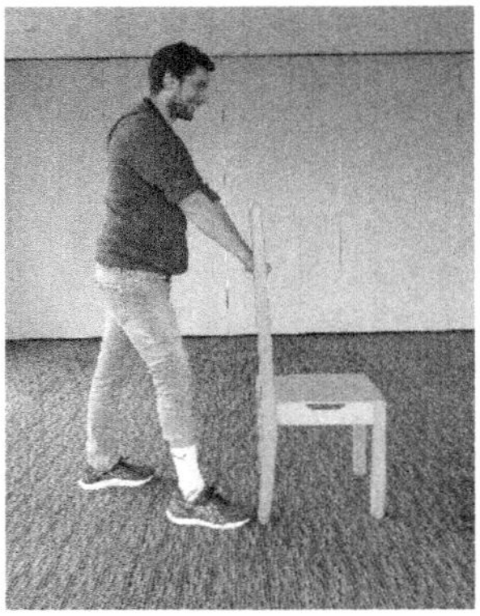

13 Foot forward with calf muscles lengthened

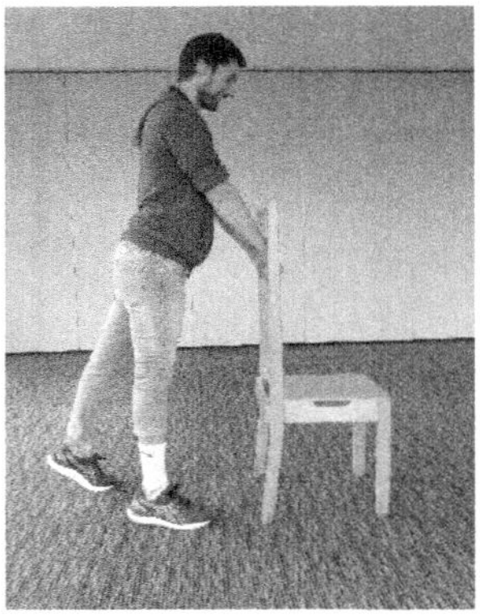

14 Ankle with leg and hip upright with stretch on the calf muscles

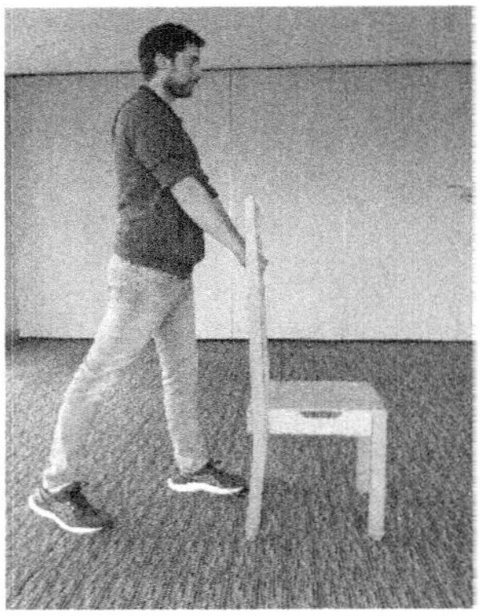

15 With increased stretch on the right hip and stretch on the right calf muscles which can stimulate the dorsiflexors muscles to lift the toes clear of the ground

Appendix 4

Advice for People with Neurological Conditions

1. Understand how your body functions and the value of stretching; also the need for moving/changing position regularly.

2. Understand what we do with our body when we relax.

3. Use the day well. Prepare for doing the things you need or want to do.

4. Keep a personal health record to help you feel in control and encourage a feeling of partnership with other members of the professional team.

How the Body Functions

POSTURE IN STANDING

Stand straight, (weight on the heels)
Head in the middle
Shoulders level
Back straight
Hips straight
Hands by the sides
(check by standing against a wall)

SITTING TO STANDING

1. Feet back, slightly apart
2. Bring hips forward to the edge of the chair
3. Lean forwards
4. Stand up
5. Stand straight (weight on the heels)

SITTING DOWN

Be aware of both feet placed near the front of the chair slightly apart (feet level – equal weightbearing, feel the chair on the back of the knees). Put hands on the arms of the chair, bend at the hips and knees, head forwards and sit down.

WALKING – Standing Straight First

1. Head up

2. Stepping forward with your unaffected foot to put the heel down first, thus stretching the affected ankle which helps to stimulate the antigravity muscles in that foot
3. Equal steps
4. Arm swing

GETTING DOWN ONTO THE FLOOR

1. Stand in front of a chair
2. Bend down to put both hands on the seat of the chair (feel the stretch on your elbows and wrists)
3. Put one knee down, put the other knee down
4. Put the hands flat on the floor to be on all fours

GETTING UP FROM THE FLOOR

1. Get onto hands and knees
2. Crawl to the nearest chair
3. Put hands on the chair with thumbs apart (to stretch your web space) Press down on the hands (to fully extend the elbow and the wrists. Lean away from the foot lifting up
4. Lift one foot up, lean forwards
5. Lift the other foot up
6. Stand up straight, head up.

BRINGING A CHAIR UP TO A TABLE

1. Stand close to the table (with the chair behind)
2. Lean forwards so that the weight is on the feet
3. Reach back for the chair
4. Pull the chair near to the table
5. And sit down

TAKING A CHAIR AWAY WHEN STANDING UP

1. Bring the feet back under the chair
2. Lean forwards and push the chair back
3. And stand up

Creating a Rhythm to the Day

1. Lying programme in bed – preparation for washing, dressing and walking.

For people with Parkinson's it is advisable that when they first go to the bathroom in the morning that they smile into the mirror and practise stretching the muscles of the face and tongue with different expressions to maintain a good social connection.

2. Fine motor movements – preparation for cooking, writing and taking money out of a purse.

3. Build in stretching throughout the day, especially standing straight, stretching the calf muscles, the wrist and the elbows.

4. Have an awareness of relaxing in a normal way. Look at the postures people adopt when you look through magazines – in everyday situations.

5. Avoid sitting still for long.

Health Record

Keep a record of the medical facts and your response to any intervention to help you have a smooth journey.

~~~~~
~~~~~

Appendix 5
Hand & Arm Rehabilitation

This Appendix shows how a person with a neurological condition that disables an upper limb can still make use of the limb and restore a degree of functionality. By using both hands clasped together, a person can use an affected hand for tasks such as drinking from a glass and opening a bottle. Such practices also prevent the person from neglecting an affected hand and arm. Before performing such tasks a brief preparatory exercise is helpful. This is shown in section 1.

1. Aim: to have two flat hands

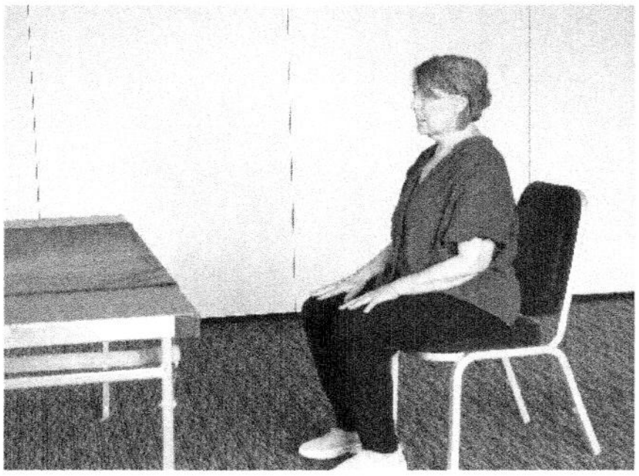

a. I sit well, feet flat under my knees, back straight, head in the middle, hands flat on my knees

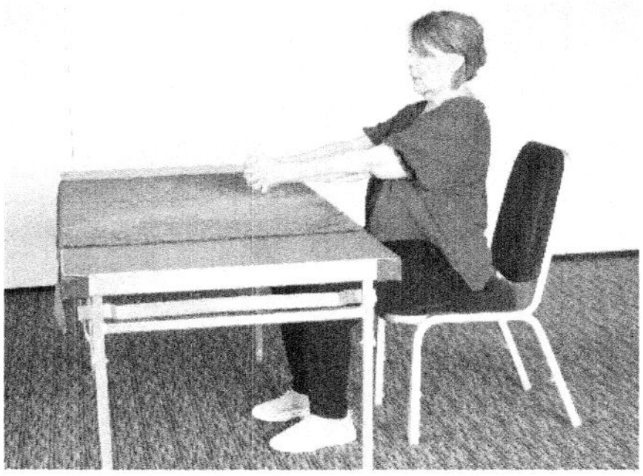

b. I clasp my hands together

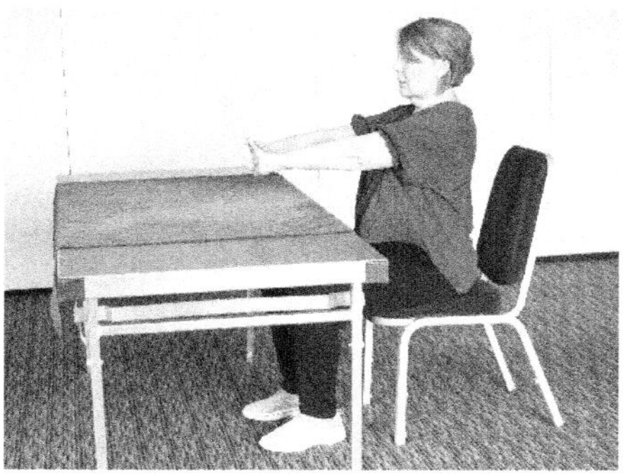

c. I turn my hands inside out

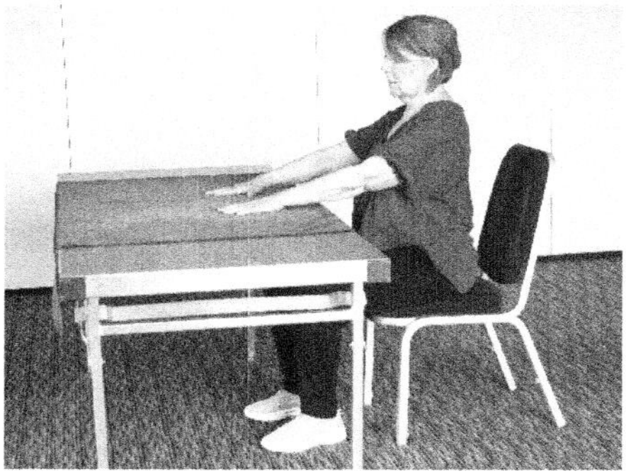

d. I separate my hands – I have two flat hands

2. Aim: to mobilise the shoulders

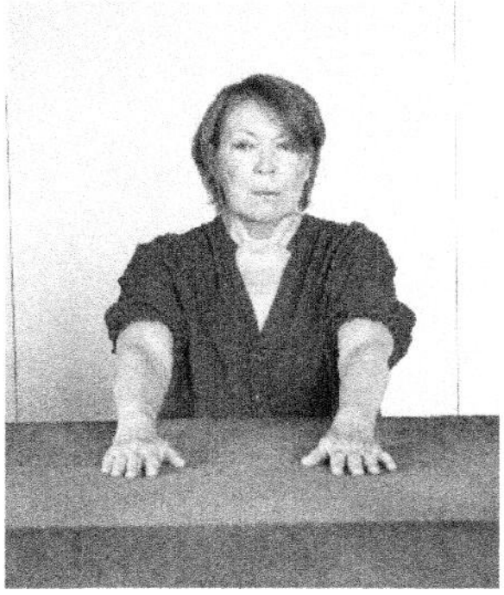

a. Starting position

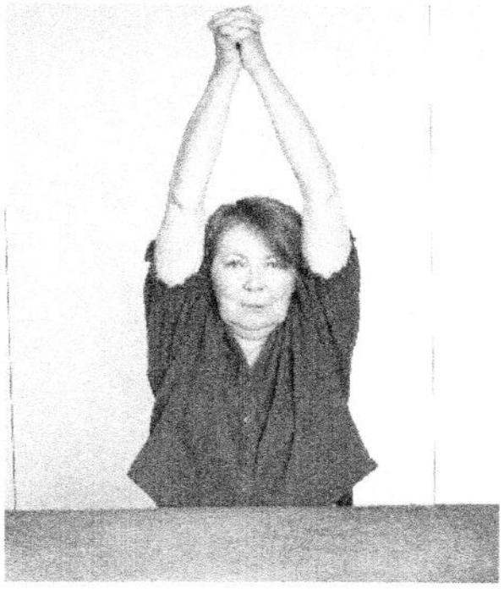

b. I lift my clasped hands above my head

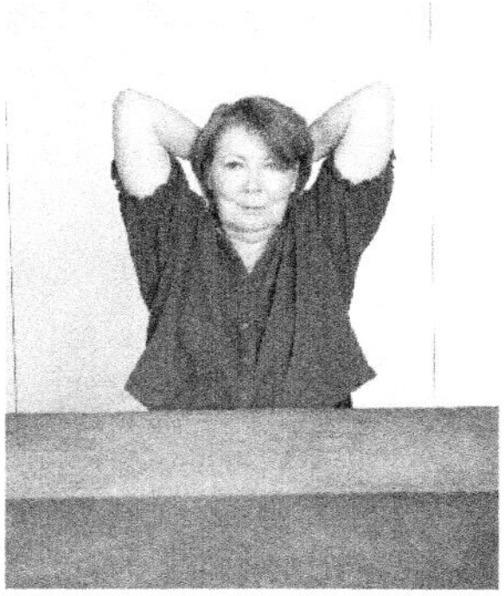

c. I put my hands behind my neck

3. Aim: to mobilise the wrists

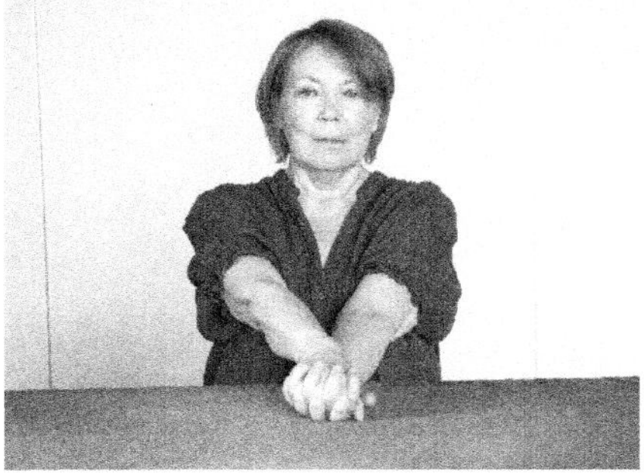

a. I put my right thumb on the table

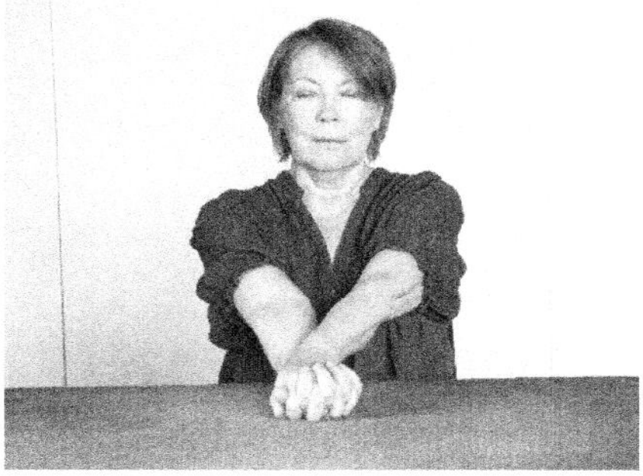

b. I put my left thumb on the table

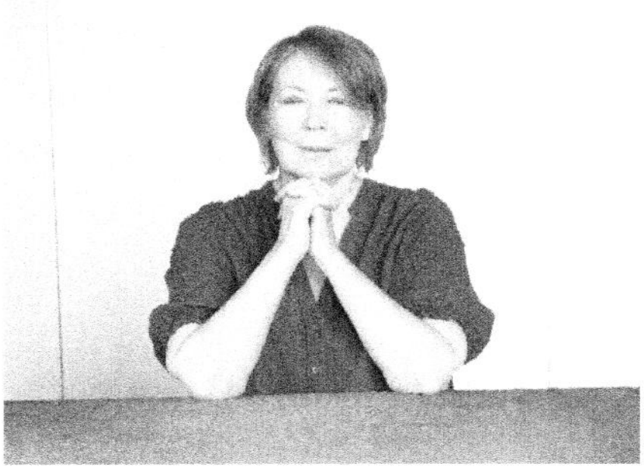

c. I put my elbows on the table with clasped hands

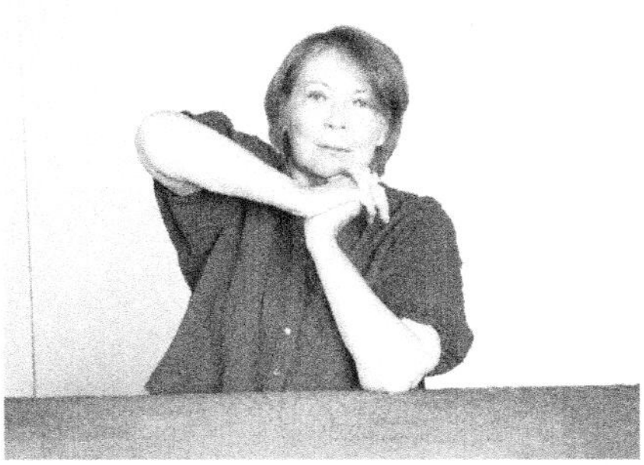

d. I lift my right elbow up pressing down to stretch my left wrist

4. Aim: to use a stick to mobilise the shoulders with preparation for grasping the stick

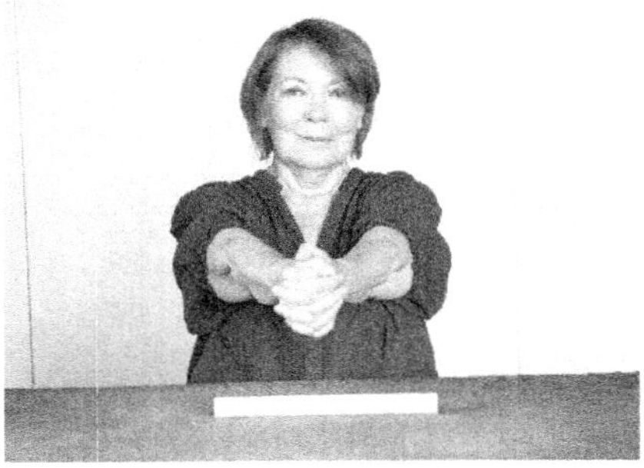

a. I clasp my hands together

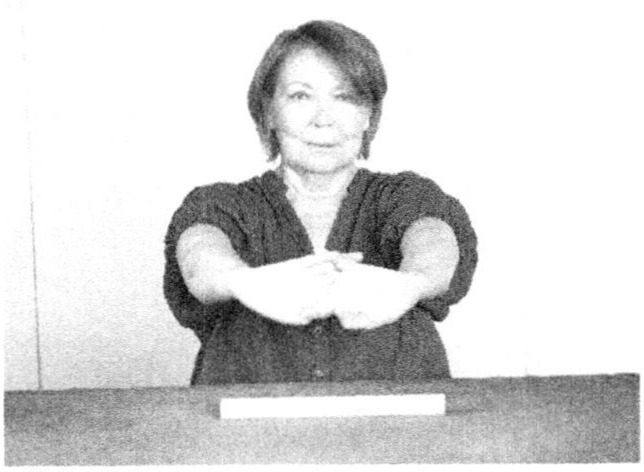

b. I turn my hands inside out

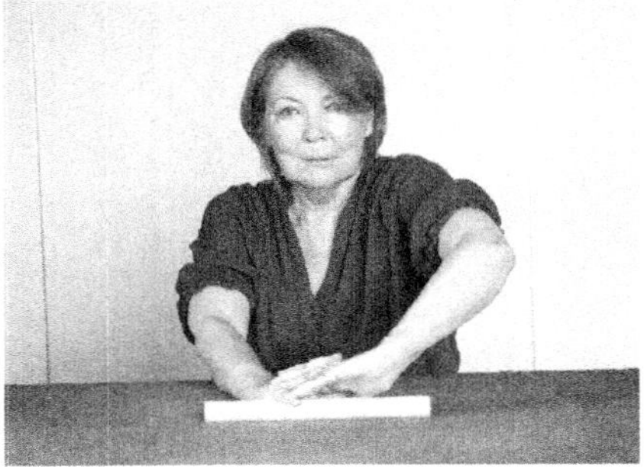

c. I place my clasped hands in the middle of the stick

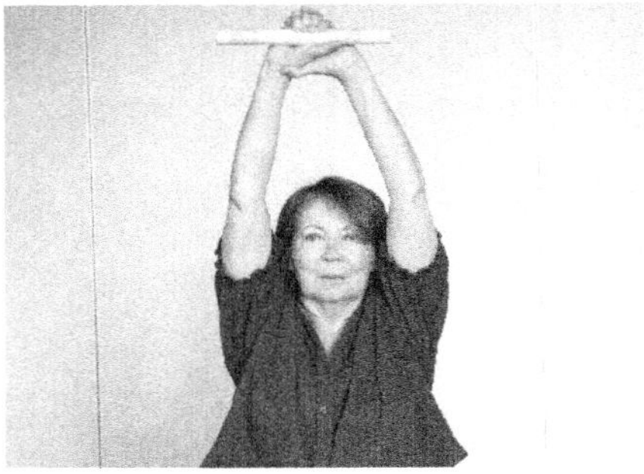

d. I lift the stick above my head

5. Aim: to mobilise the wrists using a stick

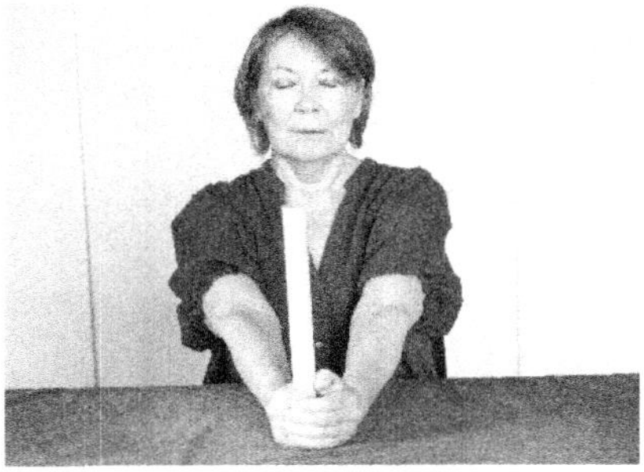

a. I hold the stick upright

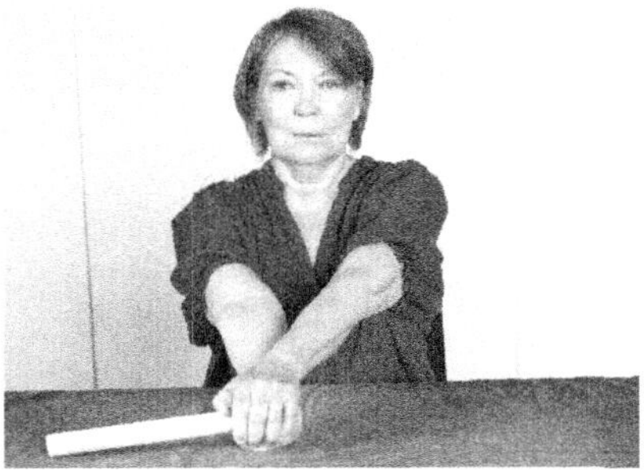

b. I twist the stick to touch the table

6. Aim: to practise grasp and release

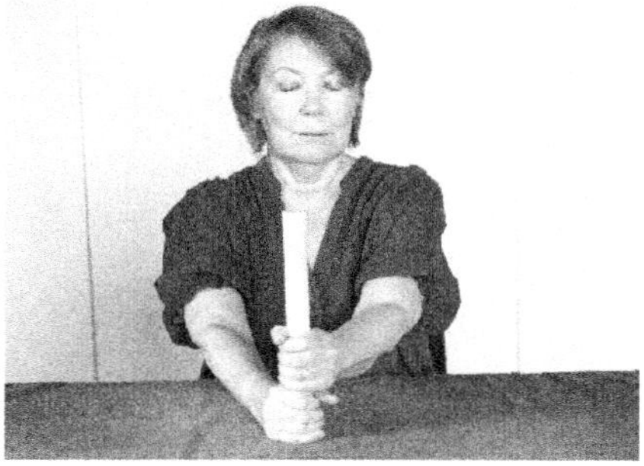

a. I put both hands at the base of the stick, one hand above the other

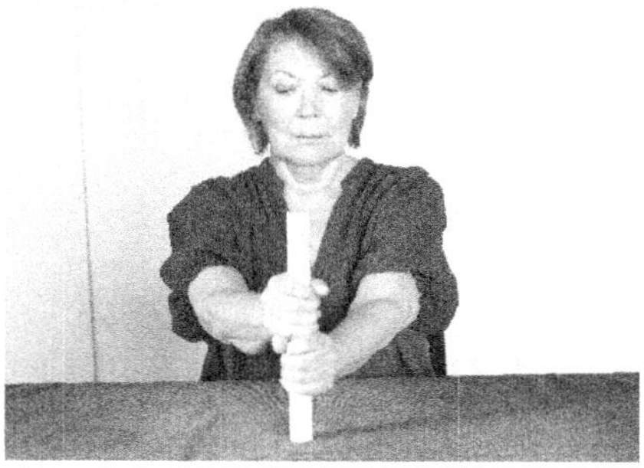

b. I let go the stick with my right hand and place it above the left

7. Aim: to use the weaker hand to fix the paper while writing

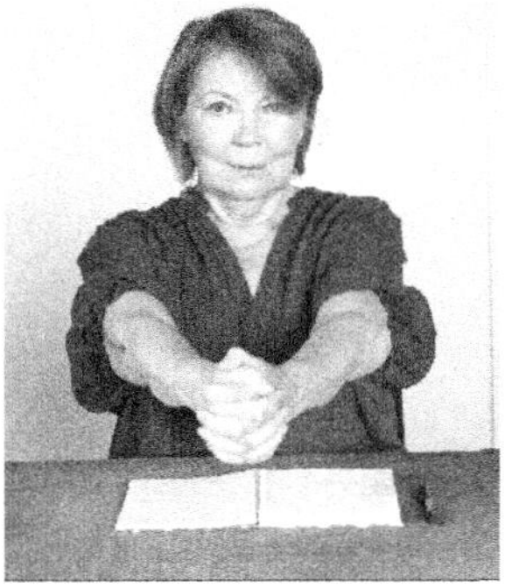

a. I clasp my hands together

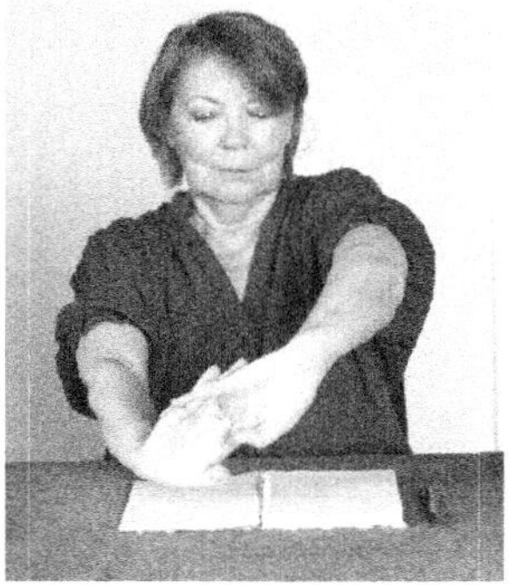

b. I turn my hands inside out

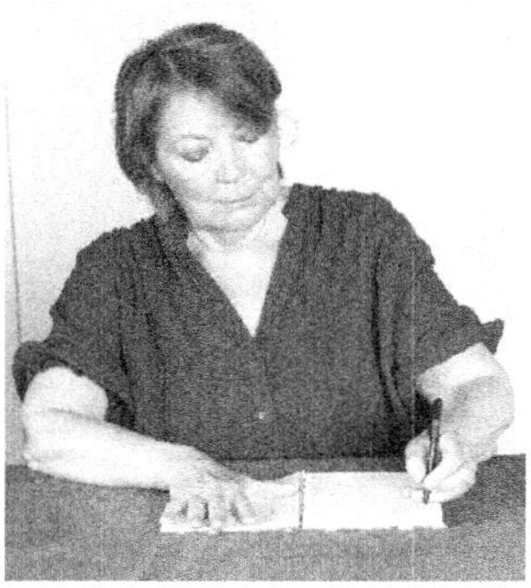

c. I place my hand on the paper

8. Aim: to hold a bottle with the affected hand to allow the unaffected hand to open the top

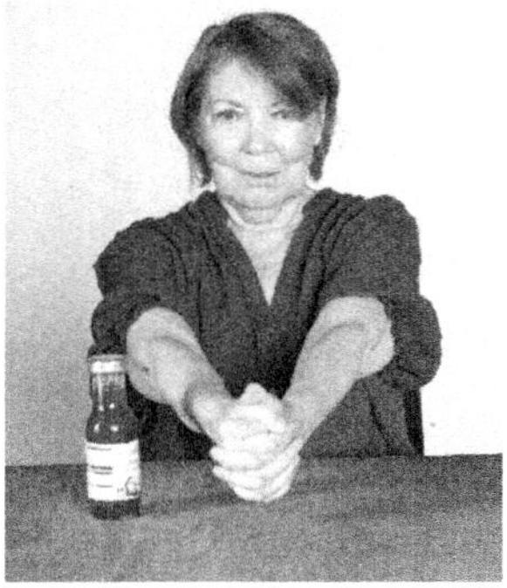

a. I clasp my hands together

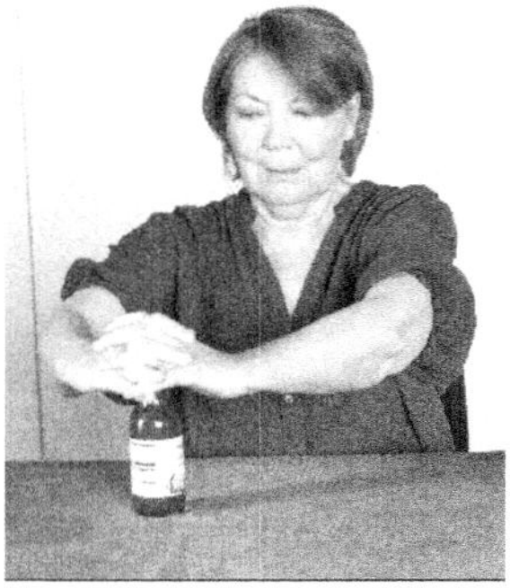

b. I place my hands over the bottle and guide the affected hand to the base. I let go the bottle with my unaffected hand

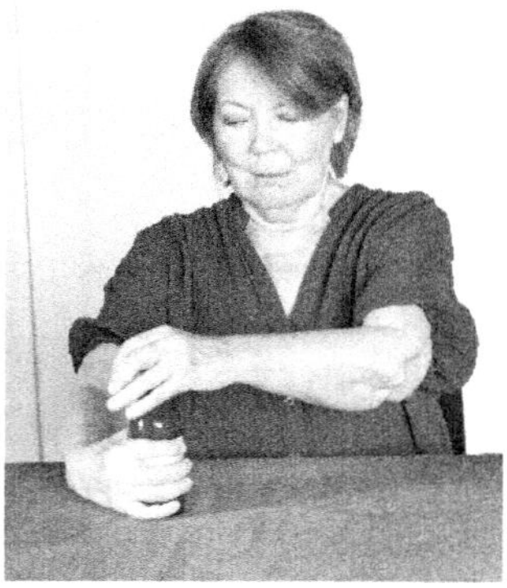

c. I take off the top

Sources of Information & Support

STROKE

Stroke Association

The Stroke Association funds research into stroke prevention, treatment and after-care. It provides a wide range of services for stroke survivors and carers across the UK, including the Stroke Recovery Service, Communication Support Service, Emotional Support Service, Exercise-based Rehabilitation Service, Post Stroke Review service, and Caring and You. https://www.stroke.org.uk/

Different Strokes

The prime objectives of the charity are to help stroke survivors of under retirement age to optimise their recovery, take control of their own lives and regain as much independence as possible by offering rehabilitative services, information and advice. https://differentstrokes.co.uk/

The ARNI Institute

The ARNI (Action for Rehabilitation from Neurological Injury) Institute is committed to teaching stroke and other acquired injury survivors to gain better action control. Their approach to stroke rehabilitation is dynamic, innovative and linked directly to the very latest neurorehabilitation evidence base. They have over 100 highly qualified independent therapists and trainers around the UK https://arni.uk.com/

PARKINSON'S

Parkinson's UK

Parkinson's UK is the largest charity funder of research into Parkinson's in the UK. It funds research for better treatments and improving the understanding of Parkinson's and its causes. It offers support and information to people affected by Parkinson's and their families and carers through a network of local groups across the UK.
https://www.parkinsons.org.uk/

European Parkinson's Disease Association (EPDA)

EPDA is the only European umbrella organisation enabling people with Parkinson’s to live a full life, while supporting the search for a cure.

https://www.epda.eu.com/

Spotlight YOPD

Spotlight YOPD is an information resource for knowledge of Young Onset Parkinson's. https://spotlightyopd.org/

BRAIN INJURY

The Brain Tumour Charity

The Brain Tumour Charity is dedicated to funding research, raising awareness of brain tumours, reducing diagnosis times and providing support and information for people with brain tumours, their families and friends. It is the largest dedicated funder of research into brain tumours globally. https://www.thebraintumourcharity.org/

Headway - The Brain Injury Association

Headway promotes understanding of all aspects of brain injury and provides information, support and services to survivors, their families and carers. In addition, Headway campaigns to reduce the incidence of brain injury. https://www.headway.org.uk/

The United Kingdom Acquired Brain Injury Forum (UKABIF)

UKABIF raises awareness of acquired brain injury in parliament and amongst policy makers. Its primary objective is to ensure that people with ABI have early access to local, specialist neurorehabilitation and follow up services in the community. https://ukabif.org.uk/

MULTIPLE SCLEROSIS

Multiple Sclerosis Society

The Multiple Sclerosis Society is the UK's largest charity for people affected by multiple sclerosis (MS). It funds research into the cure and cause of MS, campaigns for social and political change, and provides services that help people with MS and their families.
https://www.mssociety.org.uk/

Multiple Sclerosis Trust

https://mstrust.org.uk/

Overcoming MS (OMS)

Overcoming MS informs, supports, and empowers people with MS to lead a full life with evidence-based self-managed lifestyle choices. https://overcomingms.org/

OTHER

Ataxia UK

Ataxia UK is the leading national charity in the UK for people affected by any type of ataxia. Ataxia UK funds research into finding treatments and cures, and offers advice, information and support to people affected by the condition. https://www.ataxia.org.uk/

Dyscover – Specialist Aphasia Support

Dyscover provides long-term support and opportunities to people with aphasia and their families. Daily sessions are led by professional speech and language therapists and are designed to help people to adjust to living with aphasia. Dyscover helps members to develop strategies for communicating, maximise abilities and provides help and support for partners, carers and other family members. https://dyscover.org.uk/

Huntington's Disease Association

The Huntington's Disease Association supports a network of regional care advisors offering care and support to people with and at risk of Huntington's disease and their families. It also has a research programme that supports scientific and social research into HD. https://www.hda.org.uk/

Motor Neurone Disease Association (MND)

The MND Association focuses on improving access to care, research and campaigning for those people living with or affected by MND in England, Wales and Northern Ireland. https://www.mndassociation.org/

The Neurological Alliance

A coalition of more than 80 organisations working together to transform outcomes for the millions of people in England with a neurological condition. https://www.neural.org.uk/

Polio Survivors Network
https://poliosurvivorsnetwork.org.uk/new/

FOR CARERS

Carers UK
Carers UK gives expert advice and information through its telephone support service. It connects carers via carers' groups and volunteers in local communities throughout the UK and online so no-one has to care alone. Carers UK works with local authorities and other organisations to improve services for carers throughout the UK. https://www.carersuk.org/

Carers Trust
Carers Trust is a major charity for, with and about carers. It works to improve support, services and recognition for anyone living with the challenges of caring, unpaid, for a family member or friend who is ill, frail, disabled or has mental health or addiction problems. With locally based Network Partners the Trust is able to support carers in their homes through the provision of replacement care, and in the community with information, advice, emotional support, hands on practical help and access to much needed breaks. https://carers.org/

Carers First
Carers First works directly with and for carers to provide personalised information and advice. Carers First can help you find useful information through an extensive online information service. For one-to-one advice and support services, Carers First is funded to support carers living in Essex, Lincolnshire, Medway, Southend-on-Sea and London Boroughs Waltham Forest, Newham, Hackney and Haringey.
https://www.carersfirst.org.uk/

Age UK
Age UK provides services and support at a national and local level to inspire, enable and support older people. This includes help for carers looking after a partner, relative or friend who is disabled or ill due to physical or mental health. The Age UK network comprises around 125 local Age UKs reaching most of England. https://www.ageuk.org.uk/

~~~~~
~~~~~

Important Terminology

Given below are dictionary definitions of a number very important words used in this book plus a brief example of that meaning in the context of the book.

Multi-disciplinary

Combining or involving several disciplines or professional specialisations in an approach to a topic or problem.

Neurological conditions can affect many different systems of the body and for any individual there is no single discipline that combats the disease. This makes it impossible for one healthcare professional in any discipline to cover all complexities and diversities of symptoms and to deliver all options.

The disciplines needed may include neurologists, physiotherapists, occupational therapists, speech and language therapists, social workers, psychologists, counsellors, dieticians, bioengineers, and others.

Integrated

With various parts or aspects linked or coordinated.

Care is organised in a patient-centred way; every newly diagnosed patient has access to a core multi-disciplinary team; and each team has a coordinator. Care coordination is of critical importance in all disease stages as a patient's needs change. It is essential to bring the different agencies and disciplines together quickly to create an individualised care plan with the patient and the family member. All the parts are united into one whole and learn from one another.

Holistic

Treatment of the whole person, taking into account mental and social factors, rather than just the symptoms of an illness.

Support for each individual, mentally, emotionally, and physically, empowering those diagnosed to help look after themselves and to stay well for as long as possible. This not only gives patients a better quality of life but can even extend their lives. It can involve home visits, group work, activities, and outings with support for the family carers.

Ongoing
Continuing

Support is provided throughout a lifetime from diagnosis onward. The needs of the patient, which may vary in intensity and timing, are always met in order to maintain as a good a quality of life for the patient and carer as possible.

And an Important Model

Bio-Psycho-Social-Spiritual Model

All these areas interconnect and feed back to each other to preserve a stable equilibrium.

Within health care the model invites the health professional and patient to review the medical, psychology, and social background, to aid in the diagnosis and care plan.

~~~~~
~~~~~

Select Bibliography

Balchin, Tom. *Had A Stroke? Now What? Hospital to Rehabilitation and Beyond*. Bagwyn Books, 2020

Beales, David. Benning, Janice. Whitten, Helen. MacDonald, Julia. Johnson, Dr Gina. *Reclaim Health: A Recovery Strategy when doctors can't explain your symptoms*. Reclaim Health, 2019

Beales, David. *Community Care for Older People*. CRC Press, 2018

Challice, Sara. *Who Cares? – How to care for yourself whilst caring for a loved one*. Hammersmith Health Books, 2020

Costandi, Moheb. *Neuroplasticity (The MIT Press Essential Knowledge Series)*. The MIT Press, 2016

Doidge, Norman. *The Brain's Way of Healing: Remarkable Discoveries and Recoveries from the Frontiers of Neuroplasticity*. Penguin Books, 2016

----. *The Brain That Changes Itself: Stories of Personal Triumph from the Frontiers of Brain Science*. Penguin Books, 2008

Espay, Albert. Stecher, Benjamin. *Brain Fables: The Hidden History of Neurodegenerative Diseases and a Blueprint to Conquer Them*. Cambridge University Press, 2020

Fox, Michael J. *No Time Like the Future: An Optimist Considers Mortality*. Headline, 2020

----. *Lucky Man: A Memoir*. Hachette Books, 2002

Hassed, Dr Craig. *The Essence of Health: the Seven Pillars of Wellbeing*, Ebury Australia, 2008

Jelinek, Professor George. *Overcoming Multiple Sclerosis: The Evidence-Based 7 Step Recovery Program*. Allen & Unwin, 2016

Jessop, Catherine. *Pulling Through: Help for Families Navigating Life-Changing Illness*. Jessica Kingsley Publishers, 2021

Kennerly, Dr Helen. Kischka, Professor Udo. *Surviving Stroke*. Robinson, 2020

Rådestad, Linda. *STROKE REBEL: Optimizing Neuroplasticity to Beat the Odds*. Brain Rehab Distribution, 2019

Sacks, Oliver. *A Leg to Stand On.* Duckworth, 1998

Whitten, Helen. Beales, David. *Emotional Healing (for Dummies).* Wiley, 2010

~~~~~
~~~~~

NOTES

Printed in Great Britain
by Amazon

23492480R00130